Luciana Braz de Oliveira Paes
Zaida Aurora S. G. Soler

Being born in the 21st century

Luciana Braz de Oliveira Paes
Zaida Aurora S. G. Soler

Being born in the 21st century

Portrait of birth in the São Paulo Microregion of Regional Health Division XV (DRS XV)

ScienciaScripts

Cover image: www.ingimage.com

This book is a translation from the original published under ISBN 978-613-9-69271-2.

Publisher:
Sciencia Scripts
is a trademark of
Dodo Books Indian Ocean Ltd. and OmniScriptum S.R.L publishing group

120 High Road, East Finchley, London, N2 9ED, United Kingdom
Str. Armeneasca 28/1, office 1, Chisinau MD-2012, Republic of Moldova, Europe
Printed at: see last page
ISBN: 978-620-8-12953-8

Dedication

To God for always lighting my way.

To my parents Antônio and Lourdes for their encouragement, example of effort and determination, I recognise you, my immense gratitude and love.

To my husband, William, my great love who encouraged and helped, shared the sleepless nights and looked after my treasures, my daughters, in my absence.

To my daughters, even though they are so small, they have been understanding in my absence and have enlightened my thoughts in a special way, leading me to seek more knowledge. They are the reason for my joy, the purest and truest love.

To my sisters, for the love and affection that unites us.

ATo my grandparents, especially my grandmother José Braz, who always guided me and

encouraged me to study.

I love you

Special Thanks

To Prof[3] . Dr Zaida Aurora Sperli Geraldes Soler, for agreeing to guide me, for her availability and professional experience that helped me to see the paths to be taken. My eternal gratitude.

TO Dr[3] Denise Gonzalez Stellutti de Faria, for her encouragement, support and friendship.

To Dr Alfeu Accorsi Neto, for his encouragement and suggestions during the qualifying exam.

The Padre Albino Foundation, for its encouragement and collaboration in making timetables possible
to carry out this study.

Thank you

TO Dr[3] Maria Cláudia Parro for her availability, encouragement and for believing in us. my professional competence.

To Fátima Grisi Kuyumjian for her attention and willingness to help with the SINASC data collection.

To my great work friend Aline Cristina de Poli for her professional companionship.

To the teachers of the undergraduate nursing course at FIPA, Faculdades Integradas Padre Albino, for their friendship and encouragement.

To my work colleagues at the Padre Albino Hospital in Catanduva, nurses, doctors, nursing assistants and technicians for their support.

To all the women and newborns who took part in this study and for the opportunity to rethink obstetric care.

To all the teachers of the postgraduate master's programme at FAMERP, for their attention and professionalism.

To all those who have contributed to this work but have not been mentioned.

Epigraph

Maybe I didn't manage to do the best, but I fought for the best.

I'm not what I should be, but thank God I'm not what I was before.

(Marthin Luther King

SUMMARY

Summary

INTRODUCTION: Obstetric care in Brazil is a widely discussed problem, due to the absurd rates of caesarean sections and disregard for ethical and legal standards and recommendations from international and national organisations regarding care in the pregnancy-puerperal cycle. **OBJECTIVES: To** analyse the social and obstetric profile of women who gave birth between 2006 and 2014 and of caesarean sections in 2012. **METHOD:** This **is a** cross-sectional, descriptive study with a quantitative approach, carried out in a micro-region of the XV Regional Health Division in the state of São Paulo, which is a reference for 19 municipalities. It is part of the research linked to the Mother Project entitled *"Studies on humtmication in childbirth care: emphasis on the role of nurses -bptetra" - CEP Protocol 3921/2011.* The data was obtained from the Live Birth Information System (SINASC) during 2015. The chi-square test was used in the analyses to observe associations between the variables, applied at a significance level of 5%. **RESULTS:** 24247 women gave birth between 2006 and 2014; the vast majority underwent caesarean section (57.4% in the public sector and 99.3% in the private sector); 73.5% were aged between 20 and 34; 60% had a stable marital situation; 62.6% had studied between 8 and 11 years; 90.1% had seven or more antenatal appointments; 86.3% had a gestational age of 37 to 41 weeks; there was a higher occurrence of caesarean sections in 2012 (64.6% in the public sector and 98.7% in the private sector) and only 87 women assisted in the private sector had a normal birth between 2006 and 2014. Regarding the profile of women who underwent caesarean section in 2012, there was statistical significance in the higher age, higher level of education, having a partner and having more prenatal consultations. **CONCLUSION**: The data obtained in this study show that there is no scientific explanation for the abusive increase in caesarean sections in the nine years studied and that the profile of women undergoing caesarean sections has an influence on the number of caesarean sections.

socio-demographics of women from higher social classes. Thus, actions and interventions are needed to minimise the number of caesarean sections without obstetric indication, suggesting a greater involvement of obstetric nurses in the management of labour, allowing the active participation of women, complying with national and international guidelines and focusing on the humanisation of obstetric care.

Keywords: 1. caesarean section; 2. tocology; 3. normal childbirth; 4. humanised childbirth; 5. humanisation of care.

PRESENTATION

The preparation of this dissertation, on the subject of birth and obstetric care, emerged in the last eight years of professional experience, working exclusively as an obstetric nurse in a teaching hospital, witnessing an abusive increase in caesarean sections, especially in the private sector.

Over the course of my 14-year career, I've worked as a nursing assistant in various clinics at this hospital, even though I've specialised in obstetrics since 2004. In 2007 I was invited to join a group of nurses setting up an in-hospital birth centre, the aim of which was to reduce the number of caesarean sections and improve the quality of care through the work of obstetric nurses. Since then, the group has remained with three nurses and a series of difficulties have been faced, including indignation at the way in which women are led to have a caesarean section. In the face of this indignation, I realised that the way to improve care for these women, as well as to strengthen my knowledge in order to have arguments in a place with this behaviour, was to seek knowledge.

So I became interested in researching birth in the municipality of Catanduva in the 21st century, and carried out the research project with the aim of verifying the occurrence of caesarean sections in the municipality of Catanduva/SP between 2000 and 2015, identifying: time and day of birth; financing of the birth; reason for the surgical intervention; parity and social characteristics of the women; gestational age and weight of the newborns.

In carrying out this research, many difficulties were encountered, mainly with regard to the availability of data relating to the objectives regarding the financing of childbirth.

One of the objectives of the initial project was the availability of data on the indication for caesarean section, which can only be obtained from medical records, and it was not feasible to research this data at the moment due to the period planned and the number of medical records that would be collected. This variable was therefore excluded from the objective.

The period of time I wanted to collect the data from was also not possible, as the SINASC data is available from the GVE (Grupo de Vigilância Epidemiológica) from 2006 onwards. So data collection was carried out from 2006 to 2014, since the year of collection was 2015.

Due to these difficulties, the evolution of births by type of delivery in the municipality of Catanduva/SP between 2006 and 2014 was checked, taking into account sociodemographic and obstetric characteristics and the financing of childbirth, which was presented in the qualifying exam. It should be noted that the financing of childbirth is not reported in the Live Birth Certificate, so it is not available in the SINASC database. It was therefore necessary to contact the São José do Rio Preto DRSXV to find out how this data would be made available.

I received information that only data on the type of birth financed by the SUS is reported to the DRSXV in São José do Rio Preto via the Hospital Information System (SIH). So, in order to arrive at the private health result, it was necessary to make the difference between births in the SUS and the total number of births in the SINASC.

When I analysed this data, I noticed with the supervisor of this research that the highest number of caesarean sections was in 2012, so this year was used to describe and correlate the sociodemographic and obstetric characteristics of women who had their births by caesarean section in 2012 in a municipality in the interior of São Paulo.

In order to provide a better foundation for this study, I present below the theoretical bases for understanding this subject and the research problem being investigated.

CHAPTER 1

INTRODUCTION

The resolution of caesarean section births is a widely discussed problem in Brazil and in the region covered by DRS XV, since it includes municipalities with the highest caesarean section rates. As in other Brazilian locations, various issues have been raised to explain the abusive rates of caesarean sections in this region of São Paulo, especially in the private and supplementary health sectors, which disregard obstetric indications and the recommendations of the World Health Organisation. [1]

An internationally recognised indicator of the quality of childbirth care is the caesarean section rate, and the question arises as to what percentage is expected, justified or recommended.[2] In 1985, the World Health Organisation published the first reference in this regard, stating that there is no justification for rates higher than 10-15% in any country, state, region, municipality or health institution.[3]

From the 1980s onwards, caesarean section rates increased in Brazil, reaching almost 100 per cent among women treated in the private health system in the first decade of the 21st century.[3]

Recently, Ordinance No. 306, of 28 March 2016, approved the "Dzre/rzzes ãe^tewçõo ò GestazzZe: *a* operação *cecariana*", highlighting that in order to define the caesarean section rate in Brazil, the characteristics of our population must be taken into account, which presents distinctions related to a high number of previous caesarean operations, so that the adjusted reference rate for the Brazilian population generated from the instrument developed by the WHO would be between 25%-30%.[4]

Unfortunately, we don't even have such rates for normal/vaginal births. Since the monitoring of births by the Live Birth Information System (SINASC) began in 1990, there has been a progressive rise in caesarean section rates, reaching 55.7 per cent in 2012.[5] However, if we consider the caesarean section rate in the Supplementary and Private Health sector, they have been increasing and since 2005 have stabilised at between 80 and 90%. [6]

There has also been an increase in caesarean section rates among users of the Unified Health System since the late 1990s, a fact that has worried and outraged managers, professional associations, women's organisations and society in general. Among the reasons given for the increase in caesarean sections in Brazil are women's choice, the obstetrician's decision, as well as being influenced by cultural, socio-economic and obstetric factors and the way in which the delivery is paid for, whether by the private or public health subsystem.(6,7)

The issue of the route of labour has been the subject of interest in the literature, with authors from different fields of knowledge, such as medicine, nursing, social sciences, psychology, management, among others. Most of the publications found are in journals with a higher scientific impact, classified as A1, A2, B1 or B2 by the Qualis system for evaluating journals run by the Ministry of Education's Coordination for the Improvement of Higher Education Personnel (CAPES). This signals a recognition of the quality of production, given the importance of this subject. The themes that stood out in all these publications were: caesarean section as a "public health problem"; the "medical factor" in the practice of caesarean section; the question of "women's preference"; "free choice" vs. "female empowerment"; inequalities in health provision and the "commodification" of childbirth care; the socio-cultural context: status, ideology of safety and planning.(8)

The growing increase in caesarean section rates around the world and particularly in Brazil has made the birth scenario worrying. These rates began to accelerate progressively from the 1970s onwards, becoming a real epidemic and a serious public health problem.(9) Birth influences an important part of a population. Every year in Brazil there are at least three million births, around 98 per cent in hospitals, which means six million people (mothers/children) experiencing this moment.(10, 11)

In analysing the increase in the proportion of caesarean sections in various countries around the world, it was estimated that 1.5 million unnecessary caesarean sections are carried out in Latin America each year, causing around 100 maternal deaths and 40,000 cases of neonatal respiratory disease, probably increasing the occurrence of premature births and neonatal mortality.(12)

In general, the publications related to caesarean sections in Brazil address issues that have led to alarming rates and concern about the possibility of irreversibility in the short or medium term of this technocratic, medicalised and hospital-centred obstetric care model.

They also highlight: deficiencies in the professional training of doctors, who favour interventional and surgical procedures; the fact that caesarean sections are the desire or choice of the woman or her family; the vulnerability of pregnant women to the doctor and to the hunches or opinions of the people around them; and the fact that caesarean sections are usually carried out by the doctor's decision, because it is quicker and easier to fit into his or her professional schedule.[1]

In the production of knowledge and in the academic debate in the field of public health about the "decision", the "choice", the "preference" or the decision related to the route of caesarean section in Brazil, the following aspects stand out:

* Brazil has one of the highest rates of caesarean births in the world and this figure has been increasing every year, constituting a serious "public health problem"; a "national disgrace", a situation that needs to be changed and this doesn't seem to worry the medical profession;[1]

* It is often the professionals who are blamed for the increase in surgery and that the majority of Brazilian women prefer vaginal birth. There is a strong discourse that associates vaginal birth with "female empowerment" and claims that, historically, birth was an event that belonged to women; now, they have been expropriated of the right to decide, and childbirth has become a medical event, with many "unwanted caesareans" being carried out;[1,8]

* Caesarean sections have been used to satisfy a complex group of needs and justifications such as reduced pain, the desire for a tubal ligation, maternal complications and previous positive experiences of the procedure. Some research also shows a higher proportion of births by caesarean section on weekdays (compared to Sundays), as well as a higher proportion of low birth weight and increased prematurity; [13,14]

A Woman's preference for a type of birth, both in the case of caesarean section and vaginal birth, may be related to her satisfaction with a previous birth, both in previous experiences and in her family relationships and social environment.[15,16] .

* Despite the defence of many obstetricians,

the obvious increase in the percentage of caesarean sections was not associated with concomitant reductions in maternal and foetal morbidity and mortality. On the contrary, among women who underwent elective caesarean section, there was a higher incidence of haemorrhage requiring hysterectomy, anaesthetic complications, cardiopulmonary arrest, venous thromboembolism, puerperal infection, wall haematoma and prolonged hospitalisation; [(17)]

* Studies have also shown an association between elective caesarean sections and maternal morbidity and mortality, suggesting that performing this surgical procedure for low-risk births, i.e. when the indication is guided by non-clinical factors, may be contributing to keeping the maternal mortality ratio at high levels. [(2,18)]

Birth in a hospital environment has resulted in the progressive adoption of various technologies with the aim of making it safer and thus reducing maternal and perinatal morbidity and mortality. What we have seen is the materialisation of a model that considers pregnancy, labour and birth to be diseases rather than expressions of health. As a result, women and newborns are exposed to high rates of interventions, such as episiotomy, the use of oxytocin, caesarean section, nasopharyngeal aspiration and others. Even so, there is a high incidence of maternal mortality, as approximately 287,000 women die worldwide every year due to complications related to motherhood.[(1,4,19)]

In Brazil, childbirth care is mostly carried out in hospitals, mainly by doctors, with great access to and use of technology and interventions, with a gradual and staggering increase in caesarean sections. This undoubtedly shows that the supply and availability of knowledge, greater access to technology, supplies and biomedical equipment, the greater presence of qualified professionals and regulatory formulations alone do not guarantee the expected reversal of maternal and neonatal mortality.[(20)]

Interventions that should be used judiciously are routine and affect almost all the women and their children cared for in hospitals in Brazil. This excess of interventions has ended up neglecting the emotional, human and cultural aspects involved in the pregnancy/childbirth/puerperium process. What's more, it has failed to recognise that the experience lived at this time can leave positive or negative marks on women for the rest of their lives.[4]

What is evident is that complications are not decreasing but increasing, generally caused precisely by this advance, through the generalisation of its necessity and the abusive use of techniques and procedures. As a rule, obstetric practice in Brazil subjects women to rigid norms and routines that do not respect their bodies and their natural rhythm, preventing them from exercising their protagonism, which can be considered cultural iatrogeny.[20,21]

A survey on caesarean sections in 137 countries that are members of the United Nations (UN) also found that of more than 95% of births in the world in 2008, 6.2 million caesarean sections were performed without indication, half of them in China (1,976,606) and Brazil (960,687). The cost of these unnecessary caesarean sections was estimated at US$ 2.3 billion, while the cost of "necessary" caesarean sections was approximately US$ 432 million (17).

The cultural issue of birth planning is highlighted in a study that shows how the spread of the practice of birth by caesarean section, by making it possible to choose the date, has changed the dynamics of many maternity wards and hospitals. (13)

Scheduled caesarean sections have led to a decrease in births on some days and an increase on others, such as the rejection by some families of certain dates like Christmas and All Souls' Day, and the increase in surgery at times and days of the week that are more convenient for doctors.[8]

Some authors have discussed how personal and family values interfere with decisions about the route of delivery, which are made during prenatal care. Expectations regarding childbirth are permeated by cultural characteristics such as fear and not needing pain, the idea of vaginal birth as risky for the life of the mother and baby, and the attempt to plan the family's daily life around the birth event. (14)

The safety of caesarean sections is little questioned in a biomedical culture that publicises technological advances in surgery. One study defends the hypothesis that the decision to have a caesarean section early in pregnancy is related both to previous reproductive experiences, their own and those of other women in the family, and to the socio-cultural context, which is marked by fear of the pain of normal childbirth.[22]

The women interviewed revealed that the "power of decision" at the time of childbirth is strongly exercised by the doctor and that women/families are weakened by the subtle or explicit mechanisms through which medical power and the health "market" act.[1,9]

Data from the "Birth in Brazil, 2014" survey shows that women in the private sector are led to decide to have a caesarean section, while those in the public sector are not supported in their choice to have a vaginal birth at the end of their pregnancy. In both sectors, pregnant women are subjected to a model of care that makes vaginal birth a horrible experience, with the pain of labour being their greatest fear and the main reason for preferring a caesarean section.[7]

Caesarean section is influenced by the care received during prenatal care, the source of payment for the delivery and other socioeconomic factors, suggesting that in Brazil, surgical delivery is a consumer good.[23] Caesarean sections are almost universal in Brazil among women whose birth took place in the supplementary sector or was financed by direct disbursement, with a prevalence close to 90 per cent The association between high prevalence of caesarean sections and health care in the private sector occurs in practically all countries, but is nowhere near the rates achieved in Brazil.[24]

Undoubtedly, in situations of maternal and foetal risk, surgical delivery is an advance in technical and scientific medicine. However, what is being problematised here is the extent to which the indication of caesarean section may be serving more commercial interests than obstetric need.[1,24] .

The fact that caesarean sections are carried out for illegitimate reasons, the omission of information during the pregnancy-puerperium cycle, in short, the disrespect for the feelings and needs of women and families in Brazil has caused outrage, representing disguised forms of obstetric violence. [1,24,25]

One of the great gaps in health care in Brazil is the absence of a teamwork philosophy that brings results in improving health indicators, particularly in perinatal care. Many adverse outcomes related to maternal and perinatal mortality and morbidity stem from weak and disjointed teamwork. In many deaths of children and women related to complications of pregnancy and childbirth, it can be seen that the team does not act in a joint and cohesive manner and that the strong hierarchy present among its members, especially hegemony, power and cruel medical corporatism, makes it difficult and often impossible for obstetricians/nurse midwives to act in a way that contributes to improving results. [1,21]

The active incorporation of other subjects, such as obstetric nurses, obstetricians, perinatal educators, psychologists and doulas, among others, into the care team should be promoted, providing comprehensive care in line with the needs of the woman and her family. In this way, the potential of each member of the team can be fully utilised, according to their technical and legal capacities, for the benefit of the woman and the child.[1,21]

There is scientific evidence that the labour and birth care model led by obstetric nurses and midwives increases the chances of spontaneous births and reduces unnecessary interventions, without compromising the health of women and babies. This contrasts with what we see in Brazil, where only 15 per cent of births were attended by nurses, obstetric nurses/obstetricians, more often in poorer regions where there are almost no doctors.[25,26]

Faced with the problem of caesarean sections in Brazil, more is needed than policies to encourage natural childbirth. It is necessary to know the reality of the region studied, characterising the profile of women/newborns with regard to birth in 2012 and co-relating the type of birth with the sociodemographic characteristics of women and newborns so that bolder measures can be taken to limit the occurrence of unnecessary caesarean sections and at the same time humanise the obstetric care provided.[1]

In view of the above, this research has the following objectives:

CHAPTER 2

OBJECTIVES

2.1 To verify the evolution of births by type of delivery in a municipality in the interior of São Paulo between 2006 and 2014, taking into account sociodemographic characteristics and financing of childbirth.

2.2 To describe and correlate the sociodemographic characteristics of women who had a caesarean section in 2012 in this municipality.

CHAPTER 3

METHOD

3.1 Study Type and Variables

This is a cross-sectional, descriptive study with a quantitative approach, with the aim of verifying the evolution of births carried out in a DRS XV micro-region between 2006 and 2014, as well as verifying sociodemographic and obstetric characteristics among those who had a caesarean section in 2012. The variables assessed in this study were:

- relationship between schooling and mother's age group,
marital status, ethnicity;
- mother's age group and marital status;
- gestational age was related to birth weight
- birth, schooling, mother's age group, profession and number of antenatal visits;
- the weight of the newborn was associated with the mother's age group, the number of prenatal consultations and the Apgar score;
- the number of antenatal care visits was associated with
with the mother's age and schooling and with the Apgar scores at the 1st and 5th minutes;
- the type of birth was associated with age,
schooling, number of antenatal appointments, marital status and mother's ethnicity, as well as NB weight and Apgar score.

3.2 Study Area

This study was carried out in the reference municipality of a micro-region of the São Paulo State Health Department, linked to the São José do Rio Preto region and known as DRS XV. There are 19 municipalities in this region and the reference city is Catanduva, which is responsible for a large demand in public health, in the outpatient and hospital sectors, at primary, secondary and tertiary levels, as described below and shown in **Figure 1.**

Catanduva micro-region: about 42 kilometres from São José do Rio Preto, it covers 19 municipalities. The city of Catanduva has two maternity hospitals: São Domingos Hospital and Father Albino Hospital .

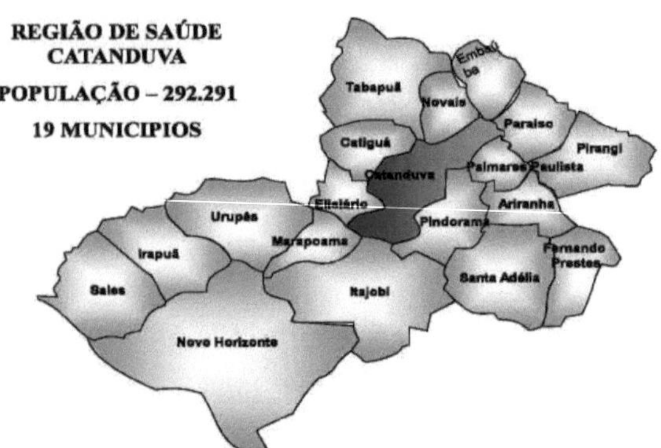

Source: Data provided by the DRS XV Directorate, 2014

Figure 1 - Geographical location of the municipalities served in Catanduva.

3.3 Reference and Data Collection Period

Births in the municipality of Catanduva from January to December 2012 were analysed, and the data was collected in 2016.

The year chosen for data collection, 2012, was chosen because it was the year with the highest number of caesarean sections in public and private healthcare in the defined data collection period (2006 to 2014).

3.4 Data Sources and Recording

Data was collected using the SINASC (Live Birth Information System) and from the São Jose do Rio Preto GVE XXIX/SP Epidemiological Surveillance Group.

We used data from SINASC, which was developed by DATASUS and implemented in 1990, based on the Declaration of Live Birth (DN). Its main objective is to provide information on the characteristics of live births, which is fundamental for establishing specific health indicators.

It is believed that the majority of births are registered in SINASC, taking into account the current legislation on vital events, including births and deaths, the Public Records Law 1, which states in Article 51 that

"Every birth that takes place on national territory must be registered at the registry office of the place where the birth took place, within fifteen days, extending to three months for places more than thirty kilometres from the *registry office*."[27]

From January 2011 onwards, the new forms were preferably used. The old variables that have changed in the way they are collected are: mother's age, mother's schooling, marital status, number of children born alive, number of children born dead, length of pregnancy, number of prenatal consultations.

3.5 Ethical issues

This study is part of the research linked to the Mother Project under the responsibility of the supervisor of this dissertation, entitled *"Eetu<as obbee a Humnizção no preparo e assistência para o nascimento: ênfase na atuação do enfermeiro obptatec" - Opinion No. 323/2011 and CEP Protocol No. 3921/2011.*

This project has not been submitted to a Research Ethics Committee *(*CEP), as it is an appendix study to the above-mentioned parent project and was carried out using databases available on the Internet from the Live Birth Information System (SINASC), which are public domain data and therefore do not require authorisation from a Research Ethics Committee involving human beings.

3.6 Data Analysis and Presentation

Statistical Analysis and Presentation of Results

In this study, the chi-square test was applied to all the analyses in order to observe possible associations between the categorised variables assessed in the study, with a significance level of 5% or ($P<0.05$) using Minitab 17 software (Minitab Inc.).

The data obtained was grouped and categorised according to similarities in order to answer the study's objective and is presented in the form of Tables.

CHAPTER 4

SCIENTIFIC MANUSCRIPTS

4.1 Manuscript 1. Birth in a Municipality in the Interior of São Paulo (20062014): until when *the* "preference" for caesarean section.

Being born in a city in the country side of São Paulo (2006-2014): how much longer will the "preference" for C-sections last.

Births in a city in the interior of São Paulo (2006-2014): when there was a "preference" for caesarean section.

MANUSCRIPT PRESENTED AT THE QUALIFYING EXAM

Luciana Braz de Oliveira Paes[1]

Obstetric nurse. Obstetric nursing coordinator at Padre Albino Hospital. Padre Albino Foundation. Catanduva, SP - Brazil.

Specialised professor. Padre Albino Integrated Colleges - FIPA. Catanduva, SP- Brazil. Master's student. São José do Rio Preto Medical School - FAMERP, Postgraduate Nursing Programme. São José do Rio Preto, SP - Brazil.

Mailing address: E-mail: luciana brazsp@hotmail.com

Zaida Aurora Sperli Geraldes Soler[2]

Obstetrician, nurse, master's, doctorate and lecturer in obstetric nursing, lecturer and supervisor of undergraduate and postgraduate courses at the Faculty of Medicine of São José do Rio Preto (FAMERP); organiser and general coordinator of the Postgraduate Course in Obstetric Nursing at FAMERP; General Coordinator of the Academic Master's Degree - Nursing Programme, FAMERP; Supervisor of the dissertation that includes this research. E-mail: zaidaaurora@gmail .com

SUMMARY

Objective: To verify the evolution of births by type of delivery, associated with social, obstetric and financing aspects, in a municipality in the interior of São Paulo. **Method:** Quantitative, descriptive, cross-sectional study, linked to the Mother Project "Studies on the birth process in São José do Rio Preto - SP and region (DRS XV)", with data obtained from

SINASC (Live Birth Information System) and SIH (SUS Hospital Information System). **Results**: there were 24,247 births; 73.46 among women aged between 20 and 34; with between 8 and 11 years of schooling (62.63%); 90.06% with more than 6 antenatal consultations; 46% publicly funded (57.49% caesarean sections); 99.34% caesarean sections in privately funded births. **Conclusion:** The data obtained is alarming, revealing that the millennium goals are not being met and that there is an urgent need to implement care measures to increase normal births, such as the work of obstetric nurses.

Keywords: 1. caesarean section; 2. normal childbirth; 3. government funding; 4. supplementary healthcare; 5. obstetric nurse.

INTRODUCTION

The increase in the occurrence of caesarean sections around the world began to be more widely discussed from the 1970s onwards, and Brazil was shamefully ranked among the top countries for the surgical resolution of childbirth. The caesarean section rate is an internationally recognised indicator of the quality of obstetric care and the World Health Organisation (WHO) published in 1985 that there is no justification for rates above 10-15%.[1,2]

In many countries, caesarean sections have high rates in the private healthcare sector, but they are nowhere near the rates achieved in Brazil.[3] Recently, Ordinance No. 306 of 28 March 2016, which approves the "Guidelines for Pregnant Women: caesarean section", took into account the characteristics and distinctions of our population, with a high number of previous caesarean operations. The WHO therefore adjusted the reference rate of caesarean sections for the Brazilian population to between 25% and 30%.[4]

Unfortunately, we don't have such rates for normal or vaginal births, at least in the private sector. Since the monitoring of births by the Live Birth Information System (SINASC) began, it has been possible to observe a progressive increase.[5] Caesarean section rates are almost universal in Brazil among women whose birth took place in the supplementary sector or was financed by direct disbursement.[6]

What is even more disheartening is the rise in caesarean section rates among SUS users, who often pay for the surgery "out of pocket". This has worried and outraged managers, professional bodies, women's organisations and society in general.[1,2,4,6-8]

In Brazil, caesarean section rates have not fallen since the 2000s, as recommended by the WHO in its Millennium Development Goals[3] . On the contrary, it has increased and is used to satisfy a complex group of needs and related justifications, such as: the obstetrician's decision, because it is quicker and easier to fit into his or her professional schedule; the vulnerability of the pregnant woman to the doctor and to the hunches or opinions of the people around her; the influence of cultural, socioeconomic, obstetric factors; the way in which the private or public health subsystem pays for childbirth; fear of the pain of labour; the desire for a tubal ligation, medical preferences, the possibility of scheduling a date and time; previous positive experiences in relation to the procedure; shortcomings in the professional training of doctors, who favour interventional and surgical procedures.[1,3,6,7,9]

Caesarean sections are influenced by the care received during prenatal care, the source of payment for the delivery and other socioeconomic factors, suggesting that in Brazil, surgical delivery is a consumer good.[9] Many interventions that should be used with discretion are routine, especially among parturients assisted in Brazilian hospitals, without considering the emotional, human and cultural aspects involved and without recognising that the experience can leave positive or negative marks for the rest of their lives.[1-6]

The preference for caesarean section is questioned, as "caesarean section on demand" is something whose causes need to be researched. It is argued that medical advice in favour of vaginal birth can have a positive effect, as can educational work aimed at the population, and obstetric nurses are highlighted as strategic professionals for humanising childbirth care and supporting women to believe in their ability to give birth.[8]

The obvious increase in the percentage of caesarean sections was not associated with concomitant reductions in maternal and foetal morbidity and mortality.[3,6] On the contrary, it was found that women who underwent elective caesarean section had a higher risk.[1,2,10] It is undeniable that in situations of maternal and foetal risk, surgical delivery is an advance in technical and scientific medicine. What is problematised is the extent to which the indication of caesarean section may be serving more commercial interests than obstetric need, causing disguised forms of obstetric violence, such as caesarean sections for illegitimate reasons, the omission of information and disrespect for women's feelings and needs. [(1,11-14)]

There is scientific evidence that the model of labour and birth care carried out by obstetric nurses/obstetricians increases the chances of spontaneous births and reduces unnecessary interventions, without compromising the health of women and babies. [12,14]

In view of the above, the **aim of** this study was **to** verify the evolution of births by type of delivery in a municipality in the interior of São Paulo between 2006 and 2014, taking into account sociodemographic and obstetric characteristics and the financing of childbirth.

METHOD

This is a descriptive, cross-sectional study, with a quantitative approach, aimed at comparing the type of birth between users of the public and private healthcare systems. It was carried out in a municipality belonging to the micro-region of the São Paulo State Health Department - DRS XV, a reference point for public and private healthcare for residents of 19 municipalities, with two hospitals with maternity wards.

The period from 2006 to 2014 was selected because only since 2006 has data been digitised and made available on the Live Births Information System (SINASC), and the year 2014 was selected because the data was collected in 2015. Also, as the data in the SINASC does not show what is public and what is private in the resolution of the birth, the Hospital Information System (SIH) was used to identify this.

This research is one of the investigations linked to the Mother Project entitled *"Studies on Humanisation in Birth Preparation and Care: Emphasis on the Role of Obstetric Nurses" - Opinion No. 323/2011 and CEP Protocol No. 3921/2011*. It is also worth clarifying that this research does not need to be approved by an Ethics Committee, in accordance with resolutions 196/1996 and 466/2012 of the CEP/CONEP system, as SINASC is a government database in the public domain and does not identify the research participants.

For statistical analysis of the data, the chi-square test was applied in order to observe possible associations between the categorised variables assessed in the study. The statistical tests were applied with a significance level of 5% or ($P<0.05$), using Minitab 17 software (Minitab Inc.). The data was grouped according to the variables defined in the research objective and the results are presented in Tables.

RESULTS

Table 1 shows data on the age range of the mothers assessed, showing that the majority were between 20 and 34 years old (1782 - 73.46%), regardless of the year assessed, with higher percentages in the 15-19 (16.05%) and 35+ (9.81%) age ranges, while there were

160 (0.65%) births in the under-15 age range.

Table 1. Percentages relating to the age group of the mothers assessed in the study. DRSXV micro-region, 2006-2014.

Track age					
Years	Under 15 years old	15 to 19 years old	20 a 34 years	35 years or older	**TOTAL**
	N	N	N	N	N and %
2006	19	464	1860	221	**2564 (10,57)**
2007	14	439	1889	194	**2536 (10,46)**
2008	20	438	1932	240	**2630 (10,85)**
2009	24	476	1990	245	**2735 (11,28)**
2010	19	396	1939	254	**2608 (10,76)**
2011	16	449	2055	318	**2838 (11,70)**
2012	15	428	2099	304	**2846 (11,74)**
2013	21	399	2032	301	**2753 (11,35)**
2014	12	405	2016	304	**2737 (11,29)**
TOTAL	**160 (0,66%)**	**3894 (16,06%)**	17812 (73,46%)	**2381 (9,82%)**	**24247 (100,00%)**

Table 2 shows the schooling of the mothers assessed in the study, and shows that regardless of the years observed, the majority of the women taking part in this study had between 8 and 11 years of schooling (1,158 - 62.64%). It can also be seen that, as the years progressed, the percentage referring to this educational level increased, from 55.42% in 2006 to 68.07% in 2014. There was a certain balance between the percentage of schooling between 4 and 7 years and 12 years or more.

Table 2. Frequencies relating to the mothers' schooling assessed in the study. DRSXV micro-region, 2006-2014.

Schooling of the mothers assessed in the study								
Years	No Inf.	Ignored	None	1 to 3 years	4 to 7 years	8 a 11	12 years and over	**TOTAL**
	N	N	N	N	N		N	**N and %**
2006	8	3	12	122	508	1421	490	**2.564 (10,57)**
2007	2	13	14	58	556	1506	387	**2.536 (10,46)**

2008	14	1	7	68	535	1606	399	**2.630 (10,85)**
2009	15	1	10	76	475	1710	448	**2.735 (11,28)**
2010	8	2	10	76	413	1628	471	**2.608 (10,76)**
2011	4	5	8	61	478	1765	517	**2.838 (11,70)**
2012	31	2	9	61	445	1855	443	**2.846 (11,74)**
2013	0	5	3	69	386	1834	456	**2.753 (11,35)**
2014	16	0	4	24	345	1863	485	**2.737 (11,29)**
TOTAL	**98 (0,40%)**	**32 (0,13%)**	**77 (0,32%)**	**615 (2,54%)**	**4141 (17,08%)**	15188 (62,64%)	**4096 (16,89%)**	**24.247 (100,00%)**

Table 3 shows the frequency of prenatal consultations carried out by the mothers assessed in the study, showing that: 21838 (90.06%) women had 7 or more prenatal consultations; for 44 (0.18%) women this information was ignored or not reported and that 139 (0.57%) women had no prenatal consultations.

Table 3. Frequencies referring to the number of prenatal consultations carried out by the mothers assessed in the study. DRSXV micro-region, 2006-2014.

Number of antenatal appointments							
Years	No Inf.	Ignored	None	1 a 3 times	4 a 6 times	7 times	**TOTAL**
	N	N	N	N	N		**N and %**
2006	3	1	20	35	176	2329	**2564 (10,57)**
2007	0	2	13	34	64	2423	**2536 (10,46)**
2008	6	2	7	14	49	2552	**2630 (10,85)**
2009	11	4	9	28	218	2465	**2735 (11,28)**
2010	2	5	13	27	188	2373	**2608 (10,76)**
2011	0	1	10	40	179	2608	**2838 (11,70)**
2012	0	5	26	68	318	2429	**2846 (11,74)**
2013	0	0	21	78	332	2322	**2753 (11,35)**
2014	0	0	20	80	300	2337	**2737 (11,29)**
TOTAL	**22 (0,09%)**	**20 (0,08%)**	**139 (0,57%)**	**404 (1,67%)**	**1824 (7,52%)**	21838 (90,06%)	**24247 (100,00%)**

The percentages relating to the mothers' gestational age are shown in Table 4 and it can be seen that the vast majority of births (20,913 - 86.24%), regardless of the year assessed, occurred when the mothers had a gestational age of 37 to 41 weeks. The subsequent gestational age with the highest number of births was 32 to 36 weeks, which ranged from 8.27% (2006) to 12.93% (2012). For the other weeks evaluated, the percentage of births was not relevant.

Table 4: Frequencies of mothers' gestational age and year of delivery. DRSXV micro-region, 2006-2014.

Gestational age									**TOTAL**
Years	No Inf.	Ignored	up to 22 weeks	22 to 27 weeks	28 to 31 weeks	32 a 36 weeks	37 a 41	42 weeks	
	N	N	N	N	N	N		N	**N and %**
2006	1	1	1	14	31	212	2265	39	**2564 (10,57)**
2007	0	7	0	13	13	221	2274	8	**2536 (10,46)**
2008	4	4	1	15	24	290	2261	31	**2630 (10,85)**
2009	6	5	1	15	28	332	2328	20	**2735 (11,28)**
2010	2	1	0	15	42	302	2244	2	**2608 (10,76)**
2011	5	1	1	14	44	332	2435	6	**2838 (11,70)**
2012	7	0	1	23	43	368	2398	6	**2846 (11,74)**
2013	0	0	0	21	46	328	2351	7	**2753 (11,35)**
2014	1	0	1	16	37	311	2357	14	**2737 (11,29)**
TOTAL	**26 (0,11%)**	**19 (0,08%)**	**6 (0,02%)**	**146 (0,60%)**	**308 (1,27%)**	**2696 (11,12%)**	20913 (86,25%)	**133 (0,55%)**	**24247 (100,00%)**

Information on the routes of normal and caesarean deliveries observed in the public and private sectors respectively is shown in Table 5:

- caesarean section deliveries were higher in both public and private healthcare;
- the percentage of caesarean sections for private sector users was significantly higher than for public health users;
- among women linked to the SUS, only in 2006 was there a higher frequency of normal births (50.46 per cent);

- there were higher rates of caesarean section in 2012 (64.65) and between 2010 and 2014 the rates were above 60 per cent;
- in the private sector, the average frequency of caesarean sections was 99.34% and the year with the highest number of normal deliveries was 2014 (30 deliveries), but with a frequency of less than 2%(1.99).

Table 5. Percentages of births by normal delivery and caesarean section in relation to the public and private spheres. DRSXV micro-region, 2006-2014.

Years	PUBLIC						PRIVATE						GRAND TOTAL	
	Normal		Caesarean section		TOTAL		Normal		Caesarean section		TOTAL			
	N	%	N	%			N	%	N	%			N	%
2006	594	50,47	583	49,53	1177	10,55	4	0,29	1383	99,71	1387	10,59	**2564**	**10,6**
2007	617	48,17	664	51,83	1281	11,48	3	0,24	1252	99,76	1255	9,59	**2536**	**10,5**
2008	581	48,91	607	51,09	1188	10,65	4	0,28	1438	99,72	1442	11,01	**2630**	**10,9**
2009	564	42,34	768	57,66	1332	11,94	2	0,14	1401	99,86	1403	10,72	**2735**	**11,3**
2010	507	40,72	738	59,28	1245	11,16	3	0,22	1360	99,78	1363	10,41	**2608**	**10,8**
2011	483	37,76	796	62,24	1279	11,47	7	0,45	1552	99,55	1559	11,91	**2838**	**11,7**
2012	426	35,35	779	64,65	1205	10,80	22	1,34	1619	98,66	1641	12,53	**2846**	**11,7**
2013	484	39,70	735	60,30	1219	10,93	12	0,78	1522	99,22	1534	11,72	**2753**	**11,4**
2014	486	39,58	742	60,42			30	1,99	1479	98,01			**2737**	**11,3**
TOTAL	**4742**	**42,51**	**6412**	**57,49**			**87**	**0,66**	**13006**	**99,34**			**24247**	**100**

DISCUSSION

The results of this study show the high occurrence of caesarean sections in the region surveyed, corroborating other research and issues debated about obstetric care in DRS XV, which favours surgical delivery and is known as the region with the most caesarean sections in Brazil. The descriptive statistics for the number of normal births and caesarean sections revealed significant differences ($P<0.001$) when comparing public and private healthcare ($P<0.001$), showing that the number of normal births was significantly higher in public healthcare (average of 526.0 births) when compared to private healthcare (average of 9.66 births). The number of caesarean deliveries (average of 1,445.1 deliveries) was significantly higher in supplementary healthcare compared to public healthcare (average of 712.44 deliveries).

With regard to sociodemographic characteristics, an increase was observed in the mothers' age group, prenatal care was carried out with a coverage of 7 or more consultations (90%); gestational age prevailed between 37 and 41 weeks (84.24%).This result makes us wonder, especially with regard to prenatal care, what kind of guidance these pregnant women are receiving with regard to the type of delivery.

These data are in line with other studies, which found that in addition to an increase in the proportion of caesarean sections in the country of around 40 per cent between 2000 and 2010, it was lower among women in the northern region of the country (42.8 per cent), among single women (42.0 per cent), among women with no schooling (25.2 per cent) and among indigenous women (16.2 per cent), with a growing tendency towards a higher probability of caesarean sections with increasing age and schooling and in the wealthier regions of the country.[5]

Another study also showed that the prevalence of caesarean section births among users of public services increased with age and schooling, and was lower among black and brown women.[15] This shows that high levels of schooling, older age, living in the wealthiest regions of the country and being white are proxies for using private services, which have high caesarean section rates when compared to public services of the same complexity.

However, it has been seen in Brazil that potential users of public services - SUS - are also above the WHO recommendations.[1-5]

Analysing deliveries in the SUS in this study, there was a decrease in the number of normal deliveries and a progressive increase in caesarean sections from 2006 to 2014. Other authors have also concluded that the high rates of caesarean sections reflect the convenience and lack of training of professionals and that, in order to justify their practice, they claim that women prefer surgery.[16] The claim that women prefer "on-demand caesarean sections" is responsible for the increase in surgery is questioned in a survey of pregnant women from low socioeconomic backgrounds, which also shows that the demand for caesarean sections is associated with women's fear of the attitudes of professionals during care and also with the desire for a tubal ligation.[17]

Therefore, "caesarean section on request" is more a consequence of a medical and institutional culture than a "real preference" on the part of women. [1720] One of the great shortcomings of health care in Brazil is the lack of teamwork to improve health indicators, revealing weak and disjointed teamwork.[13]

It was expected that the number of caesarean sections in private healthcare would be higher when compared to SUS users, but it was frightening to see the almost absolute frequency of caesarean sections among women with private health insurance. There is no discourse that can explain 87 normal births in 9 years. This means that in many months there was not even one (1) normal birth among private healthcare users, and it is also possible to assume that most of these women did not even go into labour, placing a huge burden on obstetric care.

One study found that, in the private sector, finding a doctor willing to assist with a normal birth through the health insurance scheme is not always easy, and paying the doctor directly is very expensive, even for middle-class women.[18]

On the other hand, doctors don't value the participation of obstetric nurses in the management of labour, which would relieve them of the need to monitor the dilation period, a fact that is the case in almost all developed countries and was the case in Brazil until the 1970s. This is in stark contrast to what we have found in Brazil, where only 15 per cent of births were attended by obstetric nurses/obstetricians, more often in poorer regions where there are almost no doctors. There is no criticism from the medical organisations.[12,14]

They also criticise the idea that middle- and upper-class women prefer caesarean sections to vaginal births and demand surgery.[19] For these authors, many of these surgeries are "unwanted caesareans" where women are "persuaded" at the end of their pregnancy, especially by presenting risk scenarios that are not in line with scientific evidence. It is emphasised that with the "trivialisation" of surgery, women are not surprised by its indication and adhere to the caesarean section, renouncing their initial desire for vaginal birth.[20]

This is noteworthy because these would be the women with the greatest access to health care and the lowest gestational risk, and so the caesarean section rates in this group could not be explained by medical indications. In this context, it is paradoxical that the groups in which better maternal health conditions are expected are related to higher caesarean section rates, suggesting abuse of medical technology and commercialisation in childbirth care.[21]

Comparing the number of caesarean sections and normal births in private and public healthcare in the region analysed, there is an abuse of caesarean sections and, like other authors, the issue of convenience/interest/medical power is the issue of the woman's decision/preference/choice.

The increase in pregnancies ending in caesarean section problematises women's autonomy in making decisions before doctors. Research has shown that throughout pregnancy, doctors create a scenario to justify the intervention, such as: "big baby", "narrow pelvis", "circular cord", "little fluid", "baby's position", "if the sac ruptures". In this way, women "opt" for a caesarean section for fear of being blamed for any negative outcome, and their decision is weakened by the doctors' "power of persuasion".[21]

A study of middle- and upper-class women in a private maternity hospital with a high rate of caesarean sections suggests that, even if the decision to have the operation is heavily influenced by the medical factor, women "organise" the birth of their children. This happens by transforming the event into a significant celebration of the moment of transition to motherhood, with the presence of family, filming, photography, among other things.[22]

We need to humanise birth, to give women back the leading role in childbirth, which means understanding that the woman giving birth is a human being, not a baby-making machine; showing that they are not inferior or inadequate; respecting women as the valuable beings in childbirth; that a woman's experience of giving birth makes her strong and, as a result, makes society strong. Humanised birth means putting women at the centre. It means understanding that the focus of maternity services is community-based primary care, not tertiary hospital care; that doctors and nurses must work together. Humanised birth means work based on scientific evidence and not on corporate actions aimed primarily at profit. [23]

It can be seen that the current situation regarding the resolution of childbirth in the DRS XV region studied is more critical than might have been imagined and that it is necessary to join forces to change behaviour and use strategies that will enable encouraging results, with a focus on the humanisation of childbirth.

The strategies and actions to be implemented must be based on research into social and economic issues, institutional rules, the possibilities of spaces for action, the agents involved and the determination of each one's competences, making it clear what is private and what is shared, and that the woman/family are the protagonists in this context. We are ALL supporting actors, but we are also the interlocutors in this context.

CONCLUSION

The data obtained in this study reveal significant differences in the resolution of labour between women using the public system and the private system in the DRS XV region studied, with almost all caesarean sections (99.33%) among private health users.

The alarming data obtained shows the urgency of proposing actions and interventions that achieve integrality and equality in the care provided, of breaking down corporatist medical issues, of greater inclusion of obstetric nurses, at least in the management of labour. To each their role, to all the responsibility of ethical, legal and humanistic professional behaviour.

REFERENCES:

1. Soler ZASG. CEPAHN - Centre for Humanised Birth Preparation and Assistance: a proposal for the region of São José do Rio Preto, São Paulo [livre- docência]. São José do Rio Preto: São José do Rio Preto Medical School; 2005.
2. RattnerD, Rabello-Neto DL, LanskyS, VilelaMEA,B astos MH. Caesarean sections in Brazil: situation in 2010, trends and perspectives. In: Brazil. Brasil 2011: uma análise da situação de saúde e a vigilância da saúde da mulher. Brasília: Ministry of Health; 2012. p.371-99.
3. Word Health Organisation. Appropriate technology for birth.The Lancet.1985; 8452 (2): 436-7.
4. BRAZIL. MS. Secretariat for Science, Technology and Strategic Inputs. National Commission for the Incorporation of Technologies into the SUS. Guidelines for pregnant women: caesarean section, 2016. Available at:http://conitec.gov.br accessed on 20 Jan 2016.
5. Rattner D, Moura EC. Births in Brazil: association of type of delivery with temporal and socio-demographic variables. Rev. Bras. SaúdeMatern. Infant.2016 jan/mar;16 (1): 39-47.
6. Ye J, BetránAP, VelaMG, SouzaJP, Zhang J. Searching for the optimal rate of medically necessary cesarean delivery. Birth. 2014; 41 (3): 237-44
7. Domingues RMSM, Dias MAB, Nakamura-Pereira M, Torres JA, d'Orsi E, Pereira APE, et al. Decision process for type of delivery in Brazil: from women's initial preference to the final route of delivery. Cad Saúde Pública 2014; 30 Suppl 1:S101-16.
8. Riscado LC, Jannotti CB, Barbosa RHS.The decision for the route of labour in Brazil: themes and trends in the production of collective health. Texto Contexto Enferm, 2016; 25(1).
9. Chiavegatto Filho ADP. Caesarean deliveries and the choice of birth date in the municipality of São Paulo. CiêncSaúdeColetiva. 2013 Aug; 18(8):2413-20.
10. WHO, UNICEF, UNFPA and The World Bank estimates. Geneva: World Health

Organisation, 2012. p. 59

11. Torres JA. Caesarean section and neonatal outcomes in private hospitals in Brazil: a comparative study of two different models of perinatal care. Cad. Saúde Pública 2014; 30 Sup: S220-S231.

12. Leal MdoC. Being pregnant in Brazil.Cad Saude Publica[Editorial]. 2012 Aug; 28(8): 1420-1421.

13. Andrade MAC, LimaJ.B.M.C.O.The Obstetric and Neonatal Model We Defend and Work With. Humanisation of labour and birth / Ministry of Health. State University of Ceará.Brasília: Ministry of Health, 2014. 465 p.

14. Leão MRC, Riesco MLG, Schneck CA, AngeloM.Reflections on the excess of caesarean sections in Brazil and women's autonomy. Ciênc Saúde Coletiva. 2013; 18(8):2395-400.

15. Barros AJD, Santos IS, Matijasevich A, Domingues MR,Silveira M, Barros FC, et al. Patterns of deliveries ina Brazilian birth cohort: almost universal cesarean sections for the better-off. Rev Saúde Pública. 2011; 45 (4): 635-43.

16. Faúndes A, Pádua KS, Osis MJD, Cecatti JG, Sousa MH. Opinion of Brazilian women and physicians on preference for the route of labour. Rev Saúde Pública.2004 Aug; 38(4):488-94.

17. Hotimsky S N, Rattner D, Venancio SI, BógusCM,Miranda MM. Childbirth as I see it... or childbirth as I wish it? Expectations of pregnant SUS users about childbirth and obstetric care. Cad Saúde Pública. 2002 Sep/Oct; 18(5):1303-11.

18. Barbosa GP, Giffin K, Angulo-Tuesta A, Gama AS,Chor D, D'Orsi E, et al. Caesarean section? Who wants it and under what circumstances? Cad Saúde Pública. 2003Nov/Dec; 19(6):1611-20.

19. Potter JE, Hopkins K, Faúndes A, Perpétuo I. Women's autonomy and scheduled cesarean sections in Brazil:a cautionary tale. Birth. 2008 Mar; 35(1):33-40.

20. Dias MAB, Domingues RMSM, Pereira APE, Fonseca SC, Gama SGN, Theme Filha MM et al. Women's trajectory in the definition of cesarean delivery: a case study in two units of the supplementary health system in the state of Rio de Janeiro. Ciênc. Saúde Coletiva. 2008 Sep/Oct; 13(5):1521-34.

21. Cardoso JE, Barbosa RHS. The mismatch between desire and reality: the caesarean

section industry among middle-class women in Rio de Janeiro, Brazil. Physis. 2012; 22(1): 35-52.

22. Haddad SMT, Cecatti JG. Strategies for professionals to reduce unnecessary caesarean sections in Brazil. Rev Bras Ginecol Obstet. 2011 May; 33(5):252- 62.30-O'dougherty M. Plot and irony in childbirth narrative sof middle-class.Medical Anthropology Quarterly.2013; 27(1):43-62.

23. Wagner M. Fish can't see water. The need to humanize birth.Int J Gynecol Obstet. 2001;75 (Suppl 1):S25-37. DOI:10.1016/S0020-7292(01)00519-7

4.2 Manuscript 2: Birth by caesarean section in a São Paulo micro-region: association with sociodemographic characteristics

MANUSCRIPT PRESENTED AT THE MASTER'S DEGREE DEFENCE

Luciana Braz de Oliveira Paes[1]

Obstetric nurse. Obstetric nursing coordinator at Padre Albino Hospital. Padre Albino Foundation. Catanduva, SP - Brazil.

Specialised professor. Padre Albino Integrated Colleges - FIPA. Catanduva, SP- Brazil.

Master's student. São José do Rio Preto Medical School - FAMERP, Postgraduate Programme in Nursing. São José do Rio Preto, SP - Brazil.

Mailing address: E-mail: luciana brazsp@hotmail.com

Zaida Aurora Sperli Geraldes Soler[2]

Obstetrician, nurse, master's, doctorate and lecturer in obstetric nursing, lecturer and supervisor of undergraduate and postgraduate courses at the Faculty of Medicine of São José do Rio Preto (FAMERP); organiser and general coordinator of the Postgraduate Course in Obstetric Nursing at FAMERP; General Coordinator of the Academic Master's Degree - Nursing Programme, FAMERP; Supervisor of the dissertation that includes this research. E-mail: zaidaaurora@gmail .com

SUMMARY

Birth by caesarean section in a São Paulo micro-region: association with sociodemographic characteristics.

Objective: To verify the association between the resolution of labour by caesarean section and the sociodemographic characteristics of women who gave birth in a municipality in the interior of São Paulo state in 2012. Method: Quantitative, descriptive, cross-sectional study linked to the Mother Project "Studies on the birth process in Regional Health Division XV (DRSXV)", with data obtained from the Live Birth Information System - SINASC, using the chi-square test in the statistical analysis, with a significance level of 5%. Results: 2846 live births took place in 2012 in the city studied, the majority by caesarean section (2396 - 84.2%). The majority of women who underwent caesarean section were: aged between 21 and 30 (53.7%); had between 8 and 11 years of schooling (65.9%); were married to a partner (66.4%); had seven or more antenatal consultations (87.8%) and ethnicity was not informed for 68.4% of women, followed by 24.3% of white women. There was a statistically significant difference in the number of caesarean sections performed by women who were older, had more schooling, had a partner and had more prenatal consultations. Conclusion: Sociodemographic characteristics affect the type of delivery and are a predisposing factor for caesarean sections among women from higher social classes. Keywords: 1. caesarean section; 2. tocology; 3. normal childbirth; 4. humanised childbirth; 5. humanisation of care.

INTRODUCTION

An internationally recognised indicator of the quality of obstetric care is the caesarean section rate.(1) In 1985, the World Health Organisation published the first reference for caesarean section rates, emphasising that there is no justification for any country, state, region, municipality or health institution to have rates higher than 10-15%.(2)

Recently, Ordinance No. 306 of 28 March 2016 approved the "Guidelines *for* Pregnancy *Care and* Caesarean section operations", highlighting that in order to define the caesarean section rate in Brazil, the characteristics of our population must be taken into account, which has a high number of previous caesarean operations, with the WHO setting a rate of between 25% and 30%.(3)

In many Brazilian regions there are no such rates of normal births, and it has been suggested that there are many reasons for the progressive increase in caesarean sections in Brazil: women's choice; the doctor's decision; cultural and socio-economic influences; obstetric factors; failures in prenatal care and payment, suggesting that surgical birth is a consumer good.(3-6)

Hospital birth has adopted technologies to make it safer, with the aim of reducing maternal and perinatal mortality, but on the other hand, it has allowed the realisation of a model that considers the pregnancy-puerperal cycle to be a disease rather than an expression of health. However, there is a high incidence of maternal mortality, as every year approximately 287,000 women die worldwide due to complications related to motherhood.[3,7]

One of the biggest gaps in health care in Brazil is the lack of teamwork that improves perinatal care indicators.[8,9] Research has been published all over the world that shows scientific evidence that obstetric nurses and midwives conducting labour increase the chances of spontaneous births and reduce unnecessary interventions, without compromising the health of women and babies.[8,9]

This contrasts with what we see in Brazil, where only 15 per cent of births were attended by nurses or obstetricians/obstetricians, more often in poorer regions where there are almost no doctors.[10-12]

Undoubtedly, in situations of maternal and foetal risk, surgical delivery is an advance in technical and scientific medicine. However, what is being problematised here is the extent to which the indication for caesarean section is serving medical interests.[13] Brazil is outraged by the fact that caesarean sections are carried out for illegitimate reasons, the omission of information during the pregnancy-puerperium cycle, the disregard for the feelings and needs of women and families, all of which reveal disguised forms of obstetric violence.[4,13,14]

In view of the above, the **aim of** this study was **to** verify the association between caesarean sections and the sociodemographic characteristics of women who gave birth in 2012 in a municipality in the interior of the state of São Paulo.

METHOD

This is a descriptive, cross-sectional study, with a quantitative approach, carried out in a city included in the micro-region of the São Paulo State Health Department - DRSXV, a reference for 19 municipalities.

Data was collected using the Live Birth Information System (SINASC). The variables assessed were: type of delivery; mother's age group, schooling, number of prenatal consultations, marital status, ethnicity, NB weight and Apgar score. The data was collected in 2016, considering births from January to December 2012, corresponding to the year with the highest caesarean section rates between 2006 and 2014.

This research is part of the parent project "Studies on the birth process in Regional Health Division XV (DRSXV). It is also worth clarifying that this research does not need to be approved by an Ethics Committee, in accordance with resolutions 196/1996 and 466/2012 of the CEP/CONEP system, because SINASC is a government database in the public domain and does not identify the participants.

The chi-square test was applied to the analyses in order to observe associations between the defined variables. The statistical tests were applied with a significance level of 5% ($P<0.05$), using Minitab 17 software (Minitab Inc.). The data was grouped according to the research objective variables and the results are presented in Tables.

RESULT

The type of birth was related to the following variables: mother's age group, schooling, number of antenatal appointments, marital status, ethnicity, NB weight and Apgar score.

Sample characterisation

Table 1 shows: **a** significant association in almost all the relationships observed, with only the association between the type of delivery and the mother's ethnicity ($P=0.417$) not being significant; a higher number of caesarean sections among mothers aged between 21 and 30 (53.7%); schooling between 8 and 11 years (65.2%); 7 or more prenatal consultations (85.3%) and marital status with a partner (64%). Ethnicity was not recorded for 68.4 per cent of the women, followed by 24.3 per cent of white women undergoing caesarean section.

With regard to the relationship between schooling and marital status, it was possible to observe a significant relationship ($P<0.001$) between the women assessed, who, regardless of whether or not they had a partner, had between 8 and 11 years of schooling. However, the data shows a certain tendency to suggest that there is a significant number of mothers with a partner who have 12 years or more of schooling and that mothers without a partner have between 4 and 7 years of schooling. The result is repeated for ethnicity (P<0.001), with the majority of mothers having between 8 and 11 years of schooling; however, there is a certain tendency to suggest that mothers of white ethnicity have 12 years or more of schooling, while mothers of non-white ethnicity have between 4 and 7 years of schooling.

Table 1. Association between type of delivery and maternal sociodemographic and obstetric variables. Municipality of DRSXV, 2012.

	Type of labour							
Age group	Vaginal		Caesarean section		Not informed		Total	
	N	%	N	%	N	%	N	%
10 to 14 years	2	0,4	13	0,5	0	0,0	15	0,5
15 to 20 years	**147**	**32,9**	418	17,4	1	0,03	566	19,9
21 to 30 years old	**223**	**49,9**	**1286**	**53,7**	1	0,03	1510	53,1
31 to 40 years old	73	16,3	**656**	**27,4**	1	0,03	730	25,7
41 to 50 years old	2	0,4	23	1,0	0	0,0	25	0,9
Total	447	15,7	2396	84,2	3	0,1	2846	100
Value P1	**<0,001**							
Education								
None	5	1,1	37	1,5	0	0,0	42	1,5
1 to 3 years	19	4,3	42	1,8	0	0,0	61	2,1
4 to 7 years	**128**	**28,6**	317	13,2	0	0,0	445	15,6
8 to 11 years	**273**	**61,1**	**1580**	**65,9**	2	0,07	1855	65,2
12 years or older	22	4,9	**420**	**17,5**	1	0,03	443	15,6
Total	447	15,7	2396	84,2	3	0,1	2846	100
Value P1	**<0,001**							
Antenatal appointments								
None	14	3,1	17	0,7	0	0,0	31	1,1
1 a 3	25	5,6	43	1,8	0	0,0	68	2,4
4 a 6	**86**	**19,2**	**232**	**9,7**	0	0,0	318	11,2
7 or more	**322**	**72,0**	**2104**	**87,8**	3	0,1	2429	85,3
Total	447	15,7	2396	84,2	3	0,1	2846	100
Value P1	**<0,001**							
Civil status								
With a partner	**228**	**51,0**	**1592**	**66,4**	2	0,07	1822	64,0
No mate	**217**	**48,5**	794	33,1	1	0,03	1012	35,6
Not informed	2	0,4	10	0,4	0	0,0	12	0,4
Total	447	15,7	2396	84,2	3	0,1	2846	100
Value P1	**<0,001**							
Ethnicity								
White	103	23,0	582	24,3	0	0,0	685	24,1
Not white	37	8,3	176	7,3	0	0,0	213	7,5
Not informed	307	68,7	1638	68,4	3	0,1	1948	68,4
Total	447	15,7	2396	84,2	3	0,1	2846	100
Value P1	**0,417**							

[1] P-value referring to the chi-squared test at P<0.05.

Tables 2 to 4 show only the 2396 caesarean deliveries carried out in 2012 in the municipality studied, analysing some associated maternal and newborn sociodemographic variables.

Gestational age

Gestational age was correlated with a number of variables in order to observe the presence of associations with the child's birth weight, schooling, mother's age group, profession and number of antenatal appointments **(Table 2)**:

- significant association between gestational age and schooling (P<0.001);
- the majority of mothers, regardless of gestational age, had between eight and 11 years of schooling (1,580 - 65.9%);
- there was no significant association between gestational age and the mother's age group P=0.175;
- the majority of mothers with a gestational age of 22 to 27 weeks had 4 to 6 appointments (53.8%);
- the majority of mothers with a gestational age over 27 weeks had 7 or more antenatal appointments (2103 - 87.8%);
- among mothers with gestational age between 28 and 31 weeks, 17 (51.5%) had 7 or more antenatal consultations and 13 (39.4%) had 4 to 6 consultations

Table 2. Relationship between gestational age and sociodemographic variables of women who underwent caesarean section. Municipality of DRSXV, 2012.

	Gestational age (weeks)							
Schooling (years)	22 a 27	28 a 31	32 a 36	37 a 41	42or +	Not informed	Total	
	N	N	N	N	N	N	N	%
No	0	1	3	26	0	0	30	**1,3**
informed None	0	1	3	3	0	0	7	**0,3**
1 a 3	0	0	14	28	0	0	42	**1,8**
4 a 7	2	7	51	254	2	1	317	**13,2**
8 a 11	**11**	**19**	**185**	**1358**	**3**	4	1580	**65,9**
12 or more	0	5	49	366	0	0	420	**17,5**
Total	13	33	305	2035	5	5	2396	**100**
Value P1	**<0,001**							
Age group (years)								
10 a 14	0	0	5	8	0	0	13	0,5
15 a 20	0	2	61	352	1	2	418	17,4
21 a 30	11	22	153	1096	2	2	1286	53,7

31 a 40	2	8	84	559	2	1	656	27,4
41 a 50	0	1	2	20	0	0	23	1,0
Total	13	33	305	2035	5	5	2396	100
P-value[1]	**0,175**							
No. of prenatal consultations								
None	0	0	3	10	0	1	14	0,6
1 a 3	5	2	13	22	0	1	43	1,8
4 a 6	**7**	**13**	69	140	2	1	232	9,7
7 or more	1	**17**	**220**	**1861**	**3**	2	2104	87,8
No informed	0	1	0	2	0	0	3	0,1
Total	13	33	305	2035	5	5	2396	100
P-value[1]	**<0,001**							

[1] P-value referring to the chi-squared test at P<0.05.

The association between newborn weight and maternal sociodemographic variables is shown below **(Table 3)**.

Birth weight

The results indicate (TAB.3) a significant association between gestational age and the child's birth weight (P<0.001).

The lower the gestational age, the lower the weight of the newborn. Table 3 also shows:

- regardless of the weight of the newborn, there was a higher frequency of births to mothers aged between 21 and 30;
- the percentage of births occurring was significantly higher for newborns (NB) weighing more than 1,000g and occurred more in mothers aged between 21 and 40;
- in the association between the weight of the NB and the number of prenatal consultations, the majority of mothers who gave birth to a NB weighing less than 1,000g had 4 to 6 more consultations than mothers who gave birth to a NB weighing more than 1,000g. There is a certain tendency to suggest that the lower the NB's weight, the lower the number of antenatal appointments;
- in the association between the NB's weight and the Apgar score at the 1st and 5th minutes, the result is similar for both cases; in other words, the Apgar score 8 to 10 (the highest score) exceeds 70% when the NB's weight

is above 1500 g, and exceeds 90% when it is above 2500 g. However, if the NB weighs less than 1,500g, they are more likely to have low Apgar scores than NBs weighing more than 1,500g. Therefore, the lower the NB's weight, the lower its Apgar score at both the 1st and 5th minute.

Table 3. Association between newborn weight and mother's age group, number of prenatal consultations and Apgar score of women and newborns born by caesarean section. Municipality of DRSXV, 2012.

Mother's age group	Newborn weight 0 to 999g		1000 a 1499 g		1500 a 2499 g		2500 a 2999 g		3 000a 3999 g		4000 g or more		Total	
	N	%	N	%	N	%	N	%	N	%	N	%	N	%
10 to 14 years	0	0,0	0	0,0	3	1,2	4	0,7	6	0,4	0	0,0	13	0,5
15 to 20 years	0	0,0	2	6,1	60	23,1	125	20,4	224	15,9	7	12,1	418	17,4
21 to 30 years old	**18**	**94,7**	**19**	**57,6**	**135**	**51,9**	**312**	**50,8**	**771**	**54,6**	**31**	**53,4**	1286	53,7
31 to 40 years old	1	5,3	**12**	**36,4**	**60**	**23,1**	**169**	**27,5**	**396**	**28,0**	**18**	**31,0**	656	27,4
41 to 50 years old	0	0,0	0	0,0	2	0,8	4	0,7	15	1,1	2	3,4	23	1,0
Total	19	0,8	33	1,4	260	10,9	614	25,6	1412	58,9	58	2,4	2396	100
P-value[1]	**0,007**													
No. of prenatal consultations														
1 a 3	6	31,6	1	3,0	7	2,7	18	2,9	10	0,7	1	1,7	43	1,8
4 a 6	**11**	**57,9**	11	33,3	56	21,5	55	9,0	94	6,7	5	8,6	232	9,7
7 or more	2	10,5	**20**	**60,6**	**195**	**75,0**	**537**	**87,5**	**1298**	**91,9**	**52**	**89,7**	2104	87,8
Not informed	0	0,0	1	3,0	2	0,8	4	0,7	10	0,7	0	0,0	17	0,7
Total	19	0,8	33	1,4	260	10,9	614	25,6	1412	58,9	58	2,4	2396	100
P-value[1]	**<0,001**													
Apgar 1st minute	0 to 999g		1000 to 1499g		1500 a 2499g		2500 a 2999g		3 000a 3999g		4000g or more		Total	
0 a 3	3	15,8	3	9,1	3	1,2	2	0,3	1	0,1	0	0,0	12	0,5
4 a 7	**8**	**42,1**	**13**	**39,4**	53	20,4	49	8,0	63	4,5	8	13,8	194	8,1
8 a 10	**8**	**42,1**	**17**	**51,5**	**204**	**78,5**	**563**	**91,7**	**1348**	**95,5**	**50**	**86,2**	2190	91,4
Total	19	0,8	33	1,4	260	10,9	614	25,6	1412	58,9	58	2,4	2396	100
P-value[1]	**<0,001**													
Apgar score 5th minute														
0 a 3	1	5,3	0	0,0	0	0,0	2	0,3	3	0,2	0	0,0	6	0,3
4 a 7	**6**	**31,6**	**9**	**27,3**	9	3,5	10	1,6	5	0,4	2	3,4	41	1,7
8 a 10	**12**	**63,2**	**24**	**72,7**	**251**	**96,5**	**602**	**98,0**	**1404**	**99,4**	**56**	**96,6**	2349	98,0
Total	19	0,8	33	1,4	260	10,9	614	25,6	1412	58,9	58	2,4	2396	100
P-value[1]	**<0,001**													

[1] P-value referring to the chi-squared test at P<0.05.

Number of antenatal appointments

The number of prenatal consultations was associated with the mother's age group, the mother's schooling and the Apgar scores at the 1st and 5th minutes **(Table 4)**:

- high association between the number of antenatal care visits and the mother's age group, and in the majority of cases,

regardless of age group, more mothers had 7 or more appointments;

- it is possible to observe a significant percentage of 4 to 6 consultations for mothers aged up to 14 years. This result indicates that the younger the mother, the lower the number of antenatal visits;
- the association between the number of consultations and schooling was also significant, showing that for all levels of schooling, 7 or more consultations were carried out more frequently;
- it is possible to observe a high percentage of mothers with no schooling who had a lower number of consultations (4 to 6). This suggests that a lack of schooling may be associated with fewer antenatal appointments;
- the results of the association between the number of antenatal visits and the Apgar scores at the 1st and 5th minute showed that the higher the number of visits, the higher the Apgar score. There is a certain tendency to suggest that the lower the number of prenatal visits, the lower the Apgar score. As such, prenatal care is a preponderant factor for the NB to be in good condition at birth;

Table 4. Association between the number of prenatal consultations and some sociodemographic data of mothers and newborns in births by caesarean section. Municipality of DRSXV, 2012.

	No. of prenatal consultations					
Age	None	1 a 3	4 a 6	7 or more	Total	
group mother(Years)	N	N	N	N	N	%
10 a 14	1	0	**3**	**9**	13	0,5
15 a 20	3	5	55	**355**	418	17,4
21 a 30	9	25	133	**1119**	1286	53,7
31 a 40	4	13	40	**599**	656	27,4
41 a 50	0	0	1	**22**	23	1,0
Total	17	43	232	2104	2396	100
P-value[1]	**0,002**					
Education						
Not informed	0	0	4	**26**	30	1,3
None	0	0	**3**	**4**	7	0,3

1 to 3 years	3	2	8	**29**	42	1,8
4 to 7 years	5	12	58	**242**	317	13,2
8 to 11 years	8	25	148	**1399**	1580	65,9
12 years or older	1	4	11	**404**	420	17,5
Total	17	43	232	2104	2396	100
P-value[1]	**<0,001**					
Apgar1st minute						
0 a 3	1	**3**	**3**	**5**	12	0,5
4 a 7	0	2	34	**158**	194	8,1
8 a 10	**16**	**38**	**195**	**1941**	2190	91,4
Total	17	43	232	2104	2396	100
P-value[1]	**<0,001**					
Apgar score 5th minute						
0 a 3	0	1	1	**4**	6	0,3
4 a 7	1	2	**14**	**24**	41	1,7
8 a 10	**16**	**40**	**217**	**2076**	2349	98,0
Total	17	43	232	2104	2396	100
P-value[1]	**<0,001**					

[1] P-value referring to the chi-squared test at $P<0.05$.

The type of birth was related to some of the variables studied, namely: mother's age, schooling, number of antenatal appointments, marital status, ethnicity, NB weight and Apgar score **(Table 5).**

Type of labour

The results in Table 5 indicate the presence of a significant association in almost all the relationships observed, with only the relationship between the type of birth and the mother's ethnicity (P=0.417) not being significant. Table 5 also shows:

- the relationship between the type of delivery and the mother's age group showed a higher occurrence of caesarean section in mothers aged between 21 and 30;
- there is a certain balance between the ages of mothers who have delivered vaginally, with ages between 15 and 30. As such, there is a certain tendency to suggest that younger mothers opt for vaginal delivery and older mothers opt for caesarean section;
- in the relationship between type of birth and schooling, in both cases of vaginal or caesarean birth, the majority of mothers had between 8 and 11 years of schooling. There is a certain tendency to suggest that mothers with less schooling (4 to 7 years) opt for vaginal delivery and mothers

with more schooling (12 years or more) opt for caesarean section;

• with regard to the number of appointments, the result is similar, i.e. in both cases, the mothers had 7 or more antenatal appointments. There is a tendency to consider that mothers who had between 4 and 6 appointments opted for vaginal delivery, so normal delivery may be associated with fewer prenatal appointments;

• with regard to the association between the type of birth and marital status, the vast majority of mothers who were married or in a stable union opted for caesarean section, while there was a certain balance in the choice of vaginal and caesarean sections for mothers who did not have a partner. Therefore, the lack of a partner can have a significant influence on the type of birth, in which case there is a tendency to opt for vaginal birth;

• the weight of the NB was also significantly associated with the type of delivery (P=0.024), with the lower the weight of the NB, the higher the frequency of vaginal delivery. In the majority of deliveries, newborns weighing over 1000 g showed a certain tendency towards caesarean section, accounting for over 80% of the cases assessed in this study;

• both the 1st minute and 5th minute scores were higher for NBs born by caesarean section.

Table 5. Association between type of delivery and some maternal and newborn variables, according to type of delivery. Municipality of DRSXV, 2012.

	Type of labour				
	Vaginal	Caesarean section	Not informed	Total	
Mother's age group (years)	N	N	N	N	%
10 a 14	2	13	0	15	0,5
15 a 20	**147**	418	1	566	19,9
21 a 30	**223**	**1286**	1	1510	53,1
31 a 40	73	**656**	1	730	25,7
41 a 50	2	23	0	25	0,9
Total	447	2396	3	2846	100
P-value[1]	**<0,001**				
Education					
None	5	37	0	42	1,5
1 to 3 years	19	42	0	61	2,1
4 to 7 years	**128**	317	0	445	15,6
8 to 11 years	**273**	**1580**	2	1855	65,2
12 years or older	22	**420**	1	443	15,6

Total	447	2396	3	2846	100
P-value[1]	**<0,001**				
Number of prenatal consultations					
None	14	17	0	31	1,1
1 a 3	25	43	0	68	2,4
4 a 6	**86**	**232**	0	318	11,2
7 or more	**322**	**2104**	3	2429	85,3
Total	447	2396	3	2846	100
P-value[1]	**<0,001**				
Civil status					
With a partner	**228**	**1592**	2	1822	64,0
No mate	**217**	794	1	1012	35,6
Not informed	2	10	0	12	0,4
Total	447	2396	3	2846	100
P-value[1]	**<0,001**				
Ethnicity					
White	103	582	0	685	24,1
Not white	37	176	0	213	7,5
Not informed	307	1638	3	1948	68,4
Total	447	2396	3	2846	100
P-value[1]	0,417				
NB weight (grams)					
0 a 999	11	19	0	30	1,5
1000 a 1499	8	33	0	41	2,1
1500 a 2499	50	260	0	310	15,6
2500 a 2999	130	**614**	1	745	65,2
3000 a 3999	241	**1412**	2	1655	15,6
4000 or more	7	**58**	0	65	
Total	447	2396	3	2846	100
P-value[1]	**<0,001**				
Apgar 1st. Minute					
0 a 3	9	17	0	31	1,1
4 a 7	50	43	0	68	2,4
8 a 10	385	**232**	0	318	11,2
Not informed	3	**2104**	3	2429	85,3
Total	447	2396	3	2846	100
Value P1	**<0,001**				
Apgar 5°. Minute					
0 a 3	6	6	0	12	1,1
4 a 7	15	41	0	56	2,4
8 a 10	424	**2349**	3	2776	11,2
Not informed	3	0	0	3	85,3
Total	447	2396	3	2846	100
Value P1	**<0,001**				

- 1P-value referring to the chi-square test at P<0.05.

DISCUSSION

This study showed a high occurrence of caesarean sections, corroborating research that has been debated about obstetric care in our country, which favours caesarean sections. When relating the type of delivery to the mother's age group, it was observed that caesarean sections were predominant in all age groups. In the case of adolescents and younger women, the caesarean delivery route goes beyond the women's indication and preference, jeopardising their reproductive future with successive caesareans.[15,16]

Despite the high rate of caesarean sections in adolescents, this study showed that young mothers have more vaginal deliveries and older mothers opt for caesarean sections. Data also observed in studies, which found that older women were more likely to have a caesarean section. [1,15]

When assessing the association between type of delivery and ethnicity, there was no significance (P=0.417), but it should be noted that 68.4 per cent did not have this information in the SINASC records and so it was not possible to assess it. Other studies show that white women undergo caesarean sections more often than women of other ethnicities.[16,17]

In terms of the relationship between type of birth and schooling, this study found that mothers with lower levels of schooling had more vaginal births, while those with higher levels of schooling had more caesarean births. This was shown in the "Birth in Brazil" survey, which revealed that Brazilian women with less schooling were less likely to have a caesarean section. Thus, caesarean sections are performed more often by Brazilian women with a higher standard of education and socioeconomic status, as well as using more analgesia. [1, 14,15]

It can be assumed that high levels of education, older age, living in the wealthiest regions of the country and being white are proxies for using private services, which have high caesarean section rates when compared to public services. However, in Brazil, even users of public services have also been induced to have a caesarean section, often looking for alternatives to finance their birth, in agreement with the doctor of their choice. [1]

With regard to the number of antenatal appointments, the results are similar, i.e. in this study we grouped together both the women receiving care at the SUS and those with private health insurance, and in both groups the women had 7 or more antenatal appointments. In the statistical analysis, there was a tendency to consider that mothers with 4 to 6 consultations had more vaginal deliveries. It was expected that women who had more prenatal care appointments would be more likely to have a normal/vaginal birth, but in our study, in all situations, caesarean sections were more common. Thus, what we found in the region studied is what some authors have pointed out, i.e. the greater the number of consultations, the greater the exposure to caesarean section, mainly related to consultations and delivery being carried out by the same medical professional.(16,18)

The precarious quality of existing health services, the lack of integration between prenatal care and childbirth care, as well as the increase in unnecessary caesarean sections have been the main justifications for the high maternal and neonatal morbidity and mortality in Brazil, a fact that is out of step with the evolution of access to prenatal care and hospital births.[(19)] What has been debated in Brazil is the rush to bring about the birth of children, without respect for the women in the parturition process. Contrary to what is expected when prenatal care is adequate, from the start of pregnancy care, women and their families are already "led" to a caesarean section and having more than 6 prenatal appointments does not mean that they receive information about good practices and care, quite the opposite.[(1,15,20)]

The type of birth in relation to the marital status of the women in this study showed that the majority of mothers with a partner opted for caesarean section, suggesting that single women without a partner are more likely to have a normal birth. This result is in line with other studies, which show that women with higher socioeconomic status are the ones who have more caesarean sections. These would be the women with the greatest access to healthcare and the lowest gestational risk, and so the rates of caesarean sections cannot be justified within the obstetric indications. Unfortunately, what we see in Brazil, and particularly in this group, is that the women with the best maternal health conditions and the lowest obstetric risk are those who undergo the most caesarean sections.

With regard to the weight of the newborn associated with the type of delivery, this study found that the lower the weight of the newborn, the higher the frequency of vaginal delivery, which is to be expected, as there is no way of indicating caesarean section in women with a lower gestational age and low newborn weight.

The Apgar score was associated with the type of delivery, showing that both the 1st and 5th minute scores were higher for NBs born by caesarean section. Therefore, when the newborn weighs less than 1000 g, it is expected that there will be complications related to immaturity that influence the Apgar score.

In this study, we only analysed caesarean sections and the majority took place at 39 weeks, therefore with fetal maturity. Researchers warn that babies born by elective and scheduled caesarean section, without going into labour, are at high risk of mild and severe respiratory morbidity. This is neonatal near miss morbidity, which increases as gestational age decreases, showing that labour plays an important role in lung maturation. They also point to the use of unnecessary interventions, which can harm both the mother and the unborn child.[15] The absence of physiological mechanisms for adapting to birth implies a risk for babies and makes it impossible to have early skin-to-skin contact and to start breastfeeding in the first hour of life.[20]

The data obtained in this study highlights the need to propose actions and interventions to minimise the number of caesarean sections in the micro-region without obstetric indication. We suggest, as has also been emphasised in other studies, that obstetric nurses should be more involved in the management of labour. Also, that professionals assist women in the pregnancy-puerperium cycle based on the guidelines and care protocols of international and national bodies and help women to actively participate in their childbirth, empowering them to play a leading role in the humanisation of obstetric care.

CONCLUSION

This study revealed that women are being subjected to abusive and even shameful labour in the micro-region surveyed and that sociodemographic characteristics interfere with the type of delivery, with older age, more schooling, having a partner, having prenatal care and the weight of the NB being indicative of a caesarean section being predisposing factors.

REFERENCES

1. Rattner D, Moura EC. Births in Brazil: association of type of delivery with temporal and sociodemographic variables. Rev. Bras. SaúdeMatern. Infant. 2016jan/mar;16 (1): 39-47.

2. Word Health Organisation. Appropriate technology for birth.The Lancet.1985; 8452 (2): 436-7.

3. BRAZIL. MS. Secretariat of Science, Technology and Strategic Inputs. Comissão Nacional de Incorporação de Tecnologias no SUS.Diretrizes de atenção à gestante: a operação

cesariana, 2016.Disponível em:http://conitec.gov.br acesso em 20 de jan 2016.

4. Cardoso JE, Barbosa RHS. The mismatch between desire and reality: the caesarean section industry among middle-class women in Rio de Janeiro, Brazil. Physis. 2012; 22(1): 35-52.

5. Domingues RMSM, Dias MAB, Nakamura-Pereira M, Torres JA, d'Orsi E, Pereira APE, et al. Decision process for type of delivery in Brazil: from women's initial preference to the final route of delivery. Cad Saúde Pública 2014; 30 Suppl 1:S101-16.

6. Rattner D, Rabello-Neto DL, Lansky S, Vilela MEA, Bastos MH. Caesarean sections in Brazil: situation in 2010, trends and perspectives. In: Brazil. Brazil 2011: an analysis of the health situation and women's health surveillance. Brasília: Ministry of Health; 2012. p.371-99.

7. WHO, UNICEF, UNFPA and The World Bank estimates. Geneva: World Health Organisation, 2012. p. 59

8. Soler ZASG. CEPAHN - Centre for Humanised Birth Preparation and Assistance: a proposal for the region of São José do Rio Preto, São Paulo [livre- docência]. São José do Rio Preto: São José do Rio Preto Medical School; 2005.

9. Andrade MAC, LimaJBMCO .The Obstetric and Neonatal Model We Defend and Work With. Humanisation of labour and birth / Ministry of Health. State University of Ceará.Brasília : Ministry of Health, 2014. 465 p.

10. Leal MdoC. Being pregnant in Brazil.Cad Saude Publica[Editorial]. 2012 Aug; 28(8): 1420-1421.

11. Leão MRC, Riesco MLG, Schneck CA, AngeloM.Reflections on the excess of caesarean sections in Brazil and women's autonomy. Ciênc Saúde Coletiva. 2013;18(8):2395- 400.

12. Torres JA. Caesarean section and neonatal outcomes in private hospitals in Brazil: a comparative study of two different models of perinatal care. Cad. Saúde Pública 2014; 30 Sup: S220-S231.

13. BRAZIL - Ministry of Health. Secretaria de ciência, Tecnologia e Insumos Estratégicos.Departamento de Ciência e Tecnologia.PNDS 2016- Pesquisa Nacional de Demografia e Saúde da Mulher.Brasília:Editora do Ministério da Saúde,2008,583p.

14. Domingues RMSM, Dias MAB, Nakamura-Pereira M, Torres JA, d'Orsi E, Pereira APE,

et al. Decision process for type of delivery in Brazil: from women's initial preference to the final route of delivery. Cad Saúde Pública 2014; 30 Suppl 1:S101-16

15. LEAL .M.C et al.Obstetric interventions during labour and delivery in Brazilian women at usual risk.Cad. Saúde Pública, Rio de Janeiro, 30 Sup:S17- S47, 2014.

16. Gama SGN etal.Factors associated with caesarean section among primiparous adolescents in Brazil, 2011-2012. Cad. Saúde Pública, Rio de Janeiro, 30 Sup:S117-S127, 2014.

17. D'Orsi E et al. Social inequalities and women's satisfaction with prenatal care in Brazil: a national hospital-based study. Cad. Saúde Pública, Rio de Janeiro, 30 Sup:S154-S168, 2014.

18. SZWARCWALD.C.L. et al. Estimation of the maternal mortality ratio in Brazil, 2008-2011. Cad. Saúde Pública, Rio de Janeiro, 30 Sup:S71-S83, 2014.

19. Victora CG, Aquino EM, do Carmo Leal M, Monteiro CA, Barros FC, Szwarcwald CL. Maternal andchildhealth in Brazil: progressandchallenges. Lancet 2011; 377:1863-76

20. CHAVES. R.L. Birth as a radical experience of change.Cad. Saúde Pública, Rio de Janeiro, 30 Sup:S14-S16, 2014.

CHAPTER 5

DISCUSSION

The preference for caesarean section, whether it's a medical decision or a woman's choice, its authenticity, legitimacy and even the ability to choose has been widely questioned. The "on-demand" or "indicated/induced" caesarean section is something whose causes need to be understood, sometimes even to dissuade women from this inclination.

Thus, greater attention is needed to psychological aspects, more dialogue between the woman and the professional and more information during prenatal care, arguing that medical advice in favour of vaginal birth can have a positive effect. Nurses are also mentioned as strategic professionals for humanising childbirth care and supporting women to believe in their ability to give birth. Thus, the argument is that it is important to inform women and involve other professionals in order to reduce caesarean section rates.(8)

The variables analysed in this study are discussed below.

Education

The results relating to the sample characterisation of this study showed that the majority of women whose type of delivery was a caesarean section were aged between 21 and 30, with between 8 and 11 years of schooling, except for adolescent mothers, data also observed in other national studies. Research in Brazil has shown that since 2000, there has been a reduction in the absolute number of births among women under the age of 24 and an increase in the average age of mothers, which was 25.7 years in 2007; in 2009, the proportion of live births according to the mother's age was 20% in those under 20, 54.4% in mothers between 20 and 29 and 26.7% in mothers over 30.(28)

In 2013, another study found that of the 1,8009 records that made up the study population, 2,161 (12.0 per cent) were live births to teenage mothers, 13,394 (74.4 per cent) to young adult mothers and 2,454 (13.6 per cent) to late-life mothers.(29)

With regard to schooling and marital status, a significant relationship could be observed ($P<0.001$), with the majority of mothers assessed, regardless of whether or not they had a partner, having between 8 and 11 years of schooling. A significant number of mothers with a partner had 12 years or more of schooling, while mothers without a partner had between 4 and 7 years of schooling. When schooling and ethnicity were correlated, it was observed that mothers of white ethnicity had 12 years or more of schooling, while mothers of non-white ethnicity had less schooling, between 4 and 7 years.

Similar results were observed in other studies, which found that the increase in maternal schooling has accompanied the increase in the schooling of the female population. In Brazil as a whole, 8.2 per cent of mothers of newborns in 2009 had between zero and three years of schooling, 28.7 per cent had between four and seven years and 63.1 per cent had eight years or more of schooling. (30)

Mothers' age group

The relationship between the mother's age group and marital status was statistically significant (P<0.001) as the majority of mothers aged between 10 and 20 were not in any kind of marital union, while mothers aged over 20 had a husband or partner. This result is similar to that found in another study, which found that the younger the mother, the more likely she was not to be married, so that teenage mothers were more likely to be single.(29)

Gestational age

Gestational age was correlated with a number of variables in order to see if there were any associations with the child's birth weight, schooling, mother's age group, profession and number of antenatal visits. It was observed that the lower the gestational age, the lower the weight of the newborn and that those born between 22 and 27 weeks gestational age mostly weighed less than 1000g; those born between 28 and 31 weeks gestational age weighed between 1000g and 1499g; those born between 32 and 36 weeks gestational age weighed between 1500g and 2499g and those born over 36 weeks gestational age mostly weighed more than 2500g. According to other authors, very low birth weight and gestational age under 32 weeks is associated with a high risk of neonatal death. Also, as expected, preterm births are associated with low birth weight.(29)

In this study, gestational age was significantly related to schooling (P<0.001), as most mothers, regardless of gestational age, had between 8 and 11 years of schooling.

With regard to the association between gestational age and the number of prenatal consultations ($P<0.001$), it was possible to observe that the majority of mothers with gestational age between 22 and 27 weeks had 4 to 6 consultations, while the majority of mothers with gestational age over 27 weeks had 7 or more prenatal consultations. It is worth noting that although mothers with a gestational age of 28 to 31 weeks had a higher percentage of 7 or more visits (17 cases - 51.5 %), there was a significant percentage of mothers with this gestational age who had 4 to 6 antenatal visits (13 cases - 39.4 %).

One of the indicators of access to maternal and child health services used is the number of antenatal care visits. Since 2000, there has been an increase in coverage in Brazil, with the proportion of women with no consultations falling from 4.7 per cent to 1.8 per cent between 2000 and 2009.(28)

In the same period, the proportion of women who had seven or more consultations during pregnancy increased. However, in the North and Northeast the increase in this indicator was much lower, and it can be concluded that this is an index intrinsically related to the levels of socio-economic development in these regions and the availability of and access to women's and children's health care services.(28) On the other hand, the increase in prenatal care coverage does not reflect an improvement in the quality of this care.(30)

Women at higher reproductive risk, with negative outcomes in previous pregnancies, had lower prenatal care coverage, later start of care and fewer appointments than women with no history of obstetric risk.(31) Not knowing they were pregnant was a reason reported more frequently by these women when compared to those with no reproductive risk, indicating problems in diagnosing pregnancy and in being picked up by prenatal services. Similar results have been observed in other studies and reinforce the need for services to have mechanisms in place to identify these women, who would benefit most from early and adequate follow-up.(33,34)

Other studies have shown that prenatal care coverage in Brazil is practically universal, with high rates in all regions of the country and among women of different demographic, social and reproductive characteristics.(31) .However, the adequacy of this care is still low, with prenatal care starting late and many women not attending the minimum number of appointments.(34,35) Using the current recommendation of the Stork Network, it is recommended that prenatal care be started by the 12th gestational week.[a] .gestational week.(36) When other parameters are included, such as routine examinations and guidance on childbirth and breastfeeding, it was found that less than 10 per cent of pregnant women received guidance.(31)

Newborn weight

The weight of the newborn was associated with the mother's age group, the number of antenatal visits and the Apgar score. A higher frequency of births to mothers aged between 21 and 30 was observed, with a significantly higher weight for newborns (NB) weighing more than 1000g. Studies report an increased risk of a low birth weight newborn in early pregnancy due to micronutrient deficiencies and intrauterine growth restriction, leading to alterations in the evolution of the pregnancy and foetal growth, which can also result in premature birth.(37)

There is also a higher proportion of low birth weight and premature babies among teenage and older pregnant women.(29)

The association between the weight of the NB and the number of antenatal appointments showed that the majority of mothers of NB weighing less than 1000g attended between 4 and 6 appointments, a higher number than mothers who gave birth to NB weighing more than 1000g, suggesting that the lower the weight of the NB, the lower the number of antenatal appointments.

Regarding the association between the NB's weight and the Apgar score in the 1st and 5th minutes, Apgar scores 8 to 10 exceeded 70% when the NB's weight was above 1500g, and exceeded 90% when it was above 2500g. However, if the NB weighs less than 1500g, they are more likely to have low Apgar scores when compared to NBs weighing more than 1500g. Therefore, the lower the NB's weight, the lower its Apgar score at both the 1st and 5th minute. This is in line with other studies which show that birth weight, Apgar score and gestational age are significant for neonatal morbidity and consider birth weight of less than 1500g and Apgar score of less than 7 in the 5th minute to be an indicator.(38)

Prenatal care

The number of prenatal consultations associated with the mother's age group, the mother's schooling and the Apgar scores at the 1st and 5th minutes found that there was a high association between the number of prenatal consultations and the mother's age group, and in most cases, regardless of age group, the mothers had 7 or more consultations. However, a lower number of visits (4 to 6) was observed for mothers aged 10 to 14, indicating that the younger the mother, the lower the number of antenatal visits, a similar result to another study, which found that a group of adolescents were more likely to have antenatal visits with less than four.(29)

Adolescent pregnant women, especially the very young, under 15, had a later start of care and fewer appointments, demonstrating the importance of differentiated strategies for this age group.(31) Antenatal care itself should be seen as an opportunity for guidance to prevent recurrent unplanned pregnancies in adolescents.(32)

The association between the number of consultations and schooling showed that, for all levels of schooling, 7 or more consultations were carried out more frequently. However, it is possible to observe that mothers with no schooling had a lower number of consultations (4 to 6), meaning that a lack of schooling may be associated with a lower number of prenatal consultations.

Social markers are associated with the number of antenatal care visits, which is directly proportional to maternal schooling. While only 36.9 per cent of mothers with zero to three years of schooling had seven or more appointments, 80 per cent of those with 12 or more years of schooling had seven or more appointments in 2009.(28)

The results of the association between the number of antenatal visits and the Apgar scores at the 1st and 5th minute showed that the higher the number of visits, the higher the Apgar score. There is a certain tendency to suggest that the lower the number of antenatal visits, the lower the Apgar score. Thus, prenatal care is a preponderant factor for the NB to be in good condition at birth.(39)

Maternal health factors during pregnancy influence pregnancy outcomes, and quality prenatal care helps to reduce harm to the pregnant woman and her newborn. (31)

Prenatal care in Brazil was 98.7 per cent, and over 90 per cent regardless of maternal characteristics. Lower coverage was observed among puerperal women living in the North, indigenous women, those with lower levels of schooling, those without a partner and those with a higher number of pregnancies. Women with negative previous outcomes, who did not want to become pregnant, who were dissatisfied with their current pregnancy, and who reported having tried to terminate their pregnancy also had lower coverage of prenatal care. (31)

The literature identifies various barriers to not having prenatal care or to starting it early, highlighting the social inequalities that persist in the country, with less access for those with less schooling and more pregnancies, those with less schooling and those living in the North and Northeast regions. (40,41,42)

The studies also show that the low proportion of guidance received during prenatal care highlights the insufficient role of prenatal care in preparing women for childbirth and breastfeeding. Guidance on practices to facilitate childbirth, which is very important for promoting vaginal birth, was given infrequently, and guidance on signs of risk was prioritised, reinforcing the biomedical nature of care. As for the way prenatal care is organised, it is mainly provided in public services and primary care units, with only 10.4% of the women having been followed up in hospital outpatient clinics. (31)

Prenatal care carried out by professional nurses is still restricted in the country, with a higher concentration in the North and Northeast and among indigenous women, probably due to the lower availability of doctors in these regions, particularly in inland cities. According to Decree 94.406/1987 30 on the Law on the Professional Practice of Nursing, low-risk prenatal care can be provided entirely by nurses 3. In addition, one of the guidelines for prenatal care established by the Humanisation Programme for Prenatal Care and Birth (PHPN) and the Stork Network is the participation of nurses as a member of the health team that provides direct care to women during the pregnancy-puerperal cycle. (31)

The results of studies show that prenatal care coverage in Brazil is practically universal, with high rates in all regions of the country and among women with different demographic, social and reproductive characteristics.(31) Type of delivery

The type of birth was associated with some of the variables studied: mother's age, schooling, number of antenatal appointments, marital status, ethnicity, NB weight and Apgar score.

The data analysed shows that the predominant type of delivery in adolescents was caesarean section, since in the year analysed, of the 566 deliveries, 418 were caesarean sections while 147 were normal deliveries. This high proportion was also found in national studies, considering that these are adolescents and primiparous women, access to this route of delivery goes beyond the clinical indication and the preference of women, compromising the reproductive future of adolescents with successive caesarean sections in subsequent pregnancies.(43)

The results indicate that there was no significant relationship between the type of delivery and the mother's ethnicity (P=0.417). Contrary to what was found in other national studies, where there were significant differences in the care received by black and brown women in relation to the type of delivery.(44) The relationship between the type of delivery and the mother's age group showed that there was a prevalence of caesarean deliveries by mothers aged between 21 and 30; however, there was a certain balance between the ages of mothers who had vaginal deliveries, with those aged between 15 and 30. Thus, there is a certain tendency to suggest that younger mothers opt for vaginal delivery and older mothers opt for caesarean section. Data also observed in national studies, which found that older women (> 35 years) and primiparous women were also more likely to have a caesarean section.(39)

Women aged 35 and over were more likely to have a caesarean section than adults.(29)

Ratnner also found in her study that the proportion of births by caesarean section was over 80% among women with a high level of education, and between 60 and 70% among women over 30 years of age, living in the South, of yellow and white race/colour, separated and in a stable union. As for the other variables age and schooling: women over 39 had a 42% higher prevalence of surgery than those under 20; and women with 12 or more years of schooling had a 2.34 times higher prevalence of surgical deliveries than women with no schooling.(2)

The same study also found that the proportion of caesarean sections in Brazil's regions was lower in the North (42.8%), in the indigenous population (16.2%), among women with no schooling (25.2%) and among single women (42.0%), with an increasing trend with age and schooling, and that the Centre-West region had a higher probability of caesarean sections.(2)

Barros et al found an increase in the prevalence of caesarean section births as age and schooling increased, and with regard to race/colour, the highest prevalence was found among black women and the lowest among brown women (the lowest proportion), compared to white women (the highest proportion).(45)

With regard to the relationship between the type of birth and schooling, in both cases of vaginal or caesarean birth, the majority of mothers had between 8 and 11 years of schooling; however, mothers with less schooling (4 to 7 years) had a higher incidence of vaginal birth and mothers with more schooling (12 years or more) had a higher incidence of caesarean birth, which was also shown by Leal in the Birth in Brazil survey where women without health insurance, adolescents, in the lowest categories of schooling (< 7 years of schooling) and multiparous women were less likely to have a caesarean birth. 7 years of schooling), non-white (except yellow) and multiparous women were less likely to have a caesarean section.(39)

Women with higher levels of schooling and those who gave birth financed by the private sector also had a higher proportion of caesarean sections, analgesia and episiotomy, although they were less exposed to the use of oxytocin. Other authors have already shown the value of intervention, especially caesarean sections, as a good standard of care.(39)

It can be assumed that high levels of education, older age, living in the country's wealthiest regions and being white are proxies for using private services, which historically have high caesarean section rates when compared to public services of the same complexity. However, despite the high rates in these categories, the others - potential users of the public services of the Unified Health System - are also above the WHO recommendations.(2)

Caesarean section rates were much lower among less educated and non-white women, showing that excess caesarean sections mainly affect Brazilian women with a higher standard of education, reaching 89.9 per cent in the private health sector.(7)

Caesarean section was more strongly associated with the better living conditions of adolescent primiparous women, such as adequate schooling, having health insurance and even the white skin colour of the puerperal woman.(43)

With regard to the number of consultations, the result is similar, i.e. in both cases, the mothers had 7 or more antenatal consultations, however, there is a tendency to consider that mothers who had between 4 and 6 consultations deliver vaginally. This shows that prenatal care influences women to have a caesarean section, and that greater access to healthcare is related to greater interventions.

The study that analysed the factors associated with caesarean section in primiparous women in Brazil also showed similar results, since when prenatal care was classified as adequate or more than adequate, there was a higher proportion of caesarean sections, since the greater the number of consultations, the greater the adolescents' exposure to caesarean sections. This finding was also related to the fact that women have more consultations with medical professionals, especially when the birth will be assisted by them.(43)

SINASC data shows high and growing coverage in terms of access to prenatal care and hospital births. In 2010, the proportion of live births whose mothers had more than four antenatal visits was 91 per cent in the country and ranged from 80 per cent in the North to 94 per cent in the Southeast and South.(45)

Thus, the precarious quality of existing health services, the lack of integration between prenatal care and childbirth care, as well as the increase in unnecessary caesarean sections have been the main explanatory hypotheses for the high maternal mortality rates in Brazil, which are out of step with the clearly favourable temporal evolution of access to prenatal care and hospital births.(45)

One of the most striking aspects of Brazilian obstetric practice is the rush to bring about the birth of children, with no respect for women's autonomy in the parturition process. This process begins during prenatal care when women are not informed about good practices and proper obstetric care, about the benefits of vaginal birth, and are not prepared to conduct their own labour.(39)

In this study, the number of antenatal consultations is influencing the increase in caesarean sections, which should be the opposite. Other authors in a national survey have already mentioned the importance of antenatal guidance, and what guidance Brazilian women receive, guidance on beneficial practices for labour was cited by 41.1%. Guidance on signs of onset of labour and signs of risk was mentioned more by women living in the South, and to a lesser extent by those living in the North. Guidance on beneficial practices for childbirth was more frequent in the Centre-West region, which together with the North-East had the highest proportion of guidance on breastfeeding.(31)

However, many observe that, throughout pregnancy, doctors create a scenario that justifies intervention: during prenatal consultations, risks that are more supposed than real, such as "big baby", "narrow pelvis", "circular cord", are posed to women, who "opt" for a caesarean section for fear of being blamed for any negative outcome, their decision being weakened by the "power of persuasion" of doctors.(9)

Pregnant women are also influenced in other ways, as some authors carried out a review of articles published in the best-selling women's magazines in Brazil between 1988 and 2008, and observed that the advantages of caesarean sections are cited more than the risks, strengthening the idea of the safety of the surgical procedure, which can make women pay little attention to the possible harmful effects of the surgery.(8)

The type of delivery in relation to marital status showed that the vast majority of mothers who were married or in a stable union opted for a caesarean section, and the lack of a partner can also influence the choice of vaginal delivery. In this situation we have to remember that there is a possibility that was not investigated in this study in relation to the partner and the financial situation, which suggests that the partner and a more favourable financial situation interfere in the decision of women to pay for a caesarean section.

It has been mentioned in other studies that women with a higher socioeconomic status are the ones who have the most caesarean sections. In theory, these would be women with greater access to healthcare and lower gestational risk, and so the caesarean section rates in this group could not be explained simply by medical indications. In this context, according to Freitas et al, those women who are expected to have better maternal health conditions and lower obstetric risk are related to higher caesarean section rates, suggesting an abuse of medical technology in childbirth care and therefore a criticism of the commodification of labour and birth. (9)

A study of middle- and upper-class women in a private maternity hospital with a high rate of caesarean sections suggests that even though the decision to have the operation is heavily influenced by the medical factor, women "agency" the birth of their children. This happens by transforming the event into a significant celebration of the moment of transition to motherhood, with the presence of family, filming, photography, among other things. [8]

They also criticise the idea that middle- and upper-class women prefer caesarean sections to vaginal births and demand surgery. For these authors, many of these surgeries are "unwanted caesareans" and women are "persuaded" at the end of pregnancy, especially by presenting risk charts that are not in line with scientific evidence. It is emphasised that with the "trivialisation" of surgery, women are not surprised by its indication and adhere to the caesarean section, renouncing their initial desire for vaginal birth.[28]

It is argued that doctors in the private sector believe that women are mistaken when they express their desire for a vaginal birth and, with a paternalistic attitude, "persuade" their patients that the operation provides more protection for them and their babies. It is argued that, in the private sector, women's "choice" of caesarean section is the result of a type of dialogue with the doctor in which there is little encouragement for vaginal birth and "guidance" (explicit or not) towards caesarean section. [9,22]

One study, investigating the preference for caesarean sections among women from low socio-economic backgrounds, discusses the problem of excess caesarean sections as part of a market for unnecessary interventions created by inequalities in health provision.[8]

NB weight was also significantly associated with the type of delivery (P=0.024). This association shows that the lower the weight of the newborn, the higher the frequency of vaginal delivery and the higher the weight of the newborn, the higher the frequency of caesarean delivery. Thus, the weight of the NB influences the type of delivery, and in the majority of cases, newborns weighing over 1000 g are more likely to be delivered by caesarean section, accounting for over 80% of the cases assessed.

The Apgar score was associated with the type of delivery, showing that both the 1st minute and 5th minute scores were higher for babies born by caesarean section. There is a certain tendency to suggest that children born by vaginal delivery have an Apgar score in the 0 to 3 range, making up percentages close to 50 % of occurrences. This is linked to the fact that these children weigh less than 1000g, since there is a certain tendency to suggest that the lower the weight of the NB, the greater the occurrence of vaginal delivery.

It is possible that the lower Apgar scores for vaginally delivered NBs are linked to the fact that these children weigh less than 1000 g, since there is a certain tendency to suggest that the lower the weight of the NB, the greater the occurrence of vaginal delivery. Therefore, when the NB weighs less than 1000 g, it was probably born prematurely or with complications that influenced the low Apgar score.

Therefore, when the NB weighs less than 1000g, it was probably born prematurely or with complications that influenced the low Apgar score. Therefore, this data is not similar to other studies which found that babies born by elective caesarean section, when compared to those born by vaginal delivery, had a higher risk of mild and severe respiratory morbidity, which increased as gestational age decreased. The results suggest that labour plays an important role in the child's lung maturation.(46) Those born by caesarean section had a higher rate of neonatal near miss morbidity than those born vaginally. It is possible that therapeutic caesarean sections are being carried out in cases of maternal illness, but it is also possible that iatrogenic caesarean sections, which have been associated with preterm birth, may be responsible for some cases of neonatal near miss morbidity.(38)

Similarly, other studies report that a significant proportion of the complications that can occur during labour and at the time of delivery can be reduced by appropriate obstetric care, carried out with the appropriate use of technology. On the other hand, the inappropriate use of technology or unnecessary interventions can lead to pre-judgements for the mother and her unborn child.(39)

It is therefore known that high rates of caesarean sections, most of them without a precise indication and, above all, the absence of physiological mechanisms for adapting to birth, imply a risk for the babies' adaptation. The worst outcome can be seen in the high rates of prematurity, associated with respiratory disorders, such as transient tachypnoea or hyaline membrane disease.(47)

Mainly because what is most naturally expected from a healthy pregnancy, as in the vast majority of women, is the birth of healthy children who can be cared for with little intervention. For full-term newborns, we recommend early skin-to-skin contact, starting breastfeeding in the first hour of life, rooming-in and high hospitalisation in breastfeeding.[47]

The data presented describes the situation in the region analysed and is in line with other findings in the literature that show alarming figures for caesarean sections and that sociodemographic factors can be favourable to this intervention, so maternal age, schooling, having a partner or not, and having prenatal care are characteristics that influence the type of delivery. It reflects a very worrying situation, with rates above those adapted for the Brazilian population of between 25 and 30%, thus confirming that the region analysed has high caesarean section rates.

CHAPTER 6

FINAL CONSIDERATIONS

6.1 To Reflect, Conclude and Contribute

Based on our professional experience, in-depth studies and research carried out at master's level, we believe that many changes are needed in the way we give birth and this issue deserves to be widely discussed, since women are being shamefully exposed to caesarean sections, as well as sociodemographic characteristics that interfere with the type of delivery, making some characteristics such as older age, higher education, having a partner, having prenatal care and the weight of the newborn a predisposing factor for it. Thus, women and their children are prone to unnecessary procedures that increase the risk of maternal and foetal morbidity and mortality.

There is also an urgent need to propose actions that empower women, based on scientific evidence, to give them a leading role in childbirth through encouragement and preparation during prenatal care. Interventions are needed to achieve integrality and equality in the care provided, to break down corporatist medical issues, and to increase the involvement of obstetric nurses. We can see that the current state of obstetric care in our country is very critical, but it also reveals that we need to join forces to change behaviour and use strategies that will lead to encouraging results, resulting from good professional support during pregnancy, childbirth, the puerperium and care for the newborn.

CHAPTER 7

BIBLIOGRAPHICAL REFERENCES

1-Soler ZASG. CEPAHN - Centre for Humanised Birth Preparation and Assistance: a proposal for the region of São José do Rio Preto, São Paulo [livre- docência]. São José do Rio Preto: São José do Rio Preto Medical School; 2005.

2-Rattner D, Moura EC.Births in Brazil: association between type of delivery and temporal and sociodemographic variables.Rev. Bras. SaúdeMatern. Infant. 2016jan/mar;16 (1): 39-47.

3- Word Health Organisation. Appropriate technology for birth.The Lancet.1985; 8452 (2): 436-7.

4-BRASIL. MS. Secretariat of Science, Technology and Strategic Inputs. Comissão Nacional de Incorporação de Tecnologias no SUS.Diretrizes de atenção à gestante: a operação cesariana, 2016.Disponível em:http://conitec.gov.br acesso em 20 de jan 2016.

5-Rattner D, Rabello-Neto DL, Lansky S, Vilela MEA, Bastos MH. Caesarean sections in Brazil: situation in 2010, trends and perspectives. In: Brazil. Brazil 2011: an analysis of the health situation and women's health surveillance. Brasília: Ministry of Health; 2012. p.371-99.

6-Ye J, Betrán AP, Vela MG, Souza JP, Zhang J. Searching for the optimal rate of medically necessary cesarean delivery. Birth. 2014; 41 (3): 237-44

7-Domingues RMSM, Dias MAB, Nakamura-Pereira M, Torres JA, d'Orsi E, Pereira APE, et al. Decision process for type of delivery in Brazil: from women's initial preference to the final route of delivery. Cad Saúde Pública 2014; 30 Suppl 1:S101-16.

8-Riscado LC, Jannotti CB, Barbosa RHS.The decision for the route of labour in Brazil:

themes and trends in the production of collective health. Texto Contexto Enferm, 2016; 25(1).

9-Cardoso JE, Barbosa RHS. The mismatch between desire and reality: the caesarean section industry among middle-class women in Rio de Janeiro, Brazil. Physis. 2012; 22(1): 35-52.

10-BRAZIL. MS/SVS/DASIS. Live births-Brazil. Birth to mother by region. Information System on Live Births-SINASC, 2013. Available at: http://tabnet.datasus.gov.br/cgi/tabcgi.exe?sinasc/cnv/nvuf.deff>. Accessed on 20 December 2015

11-BRASIL. Ministry of Health. Secretariat of Science, Technology and Strategic Inputs. Department of Science and Technology.PNDS 2016- National Survey of Demography and Women's Health.Brasília:Editora do Ministério da Saúde,2008,583p.

12-Hofelmann DA. Temporal trend of caesarean deliveries in Brazil and its regions: 1994 to 2009. Epidemiol. Serv. Saúde 2012; 21(4): 561-568.

13-Chiavegatto Filho ADP. Caesarean deliveries and the choice of birth date in the municipality of São Paulo. Ciênc Saúde Coletiva. 2013 Aug; 18(8):2413-20

14-Pires D, Fertonani HP, ConillEM, Matos TA, Cordova FP, Mazur CS. The influence of professional health care on the choice of type of delivery: a socio-anthropological look at Brazilian supplementary health care. RevBras Saúde Mater Infant. 2010 Apr-Jun; 10(2):191-7.

15-Ferreira LA, Silva JAJ, Zuffi FB, Mauzalto ACM, LeiteCP, Nunes JS. Expectations of pregnant women regarding childbirth.RevPesq: Cuid Fundam Online. 2013 Apr-May

[access 2016Feb4]; 5(2):3692-7. Available at: http://saudepublica.bvs.br/pesquisa/resource/pt/bde-24529

16-Pimenta LF, Ressel LB, Stumm KE. The cultural construction of the birth process.J Res: Fundam Care Online. 2013 Oct-Dec [access 2016 Feb. 4]; 5(4):591- 8. Available at: http://pesquisa.bvs.br/brasil/resource/pt/bde-24959.

17-Marcolin AC. Until when will Brazil be known as the country of caesarean sections [Editorial].Rev.Bras.ginecol.obstet.2014; 36 (7): 283-289.

18-The American College of Obstetricians and Gynecologists. Cesarean delivery on maternal request. Washington: American College of Obstetricians and Gynecologists; 2013. [access in Feb 2016]. Available at: http://www.acog.org/ResourcesAndPublications/Committee-Opinions/Committee- on-Obstetric-Practice/Cesarean-Delivery-on-Maternal-Request.

19-WHO, UNICEF, UNFPA and The World Bank estimates. Geneva: World Health Organisation, 2012. p. 59.

20-Pasche DF, Vilela MEdeA, Martins CP. Humanisation of labour and birth care in Brazil: a prerequisite for a new ethic in management and care. Revista Tempus Actas Saúde Coletiva, Brasília, v. 4, n. 4, 2010.

21-Andrade MAC, LimaJBMCO .The Obstetric and Neonatal Model We Defend and Work With. Humanisation of labour and birth / Ministry of Health. State University of Ceará.Brasília : Ministry of Health, 2014. 465 p.

22-Dias MAB, Domingues RMSM, Pereira APE, Fonseca SC, Gama SGN, Theme Filha MM et al. Women's journeys towards caesarean section: a case study

in two units of the supplementary health system in the state of Rio de Janeiro. Ciênc. Saúde Coletiva. 2008 Sep/Oct; 13(5):1521-34.

23-Gama SGN. et al. Factors associated with caesarean section among primiparous adolescents in Brazil. Cad. Saúde Pública, 2014; 30 Sup:S117-S127

24-Torres JA. Caesarean section and neonatal outcomes in private hospitals in Brazil: a comparative study of two different models of perinatal care. Cad. Saúde Pública 2014; 30 Sup: S220-S231.

25-Leal MdoC. Being pregnant in Brazil. CadSaude Publica [Editorial]. 2012 Aug; 28(8): 1420-1421.

26-Leão MRC, Riesco MLG, Schneck CA, AngeloM.Reflections on the excess of caesarean sections in Brazil and women's autonomy. Ciênc Saúde Coletiva. 2013;18(8):2395- 400.

27-Brazil. Ministry of Health. Health Surveillance Secretariat. Department of Health Situation Analysis. Manual of Instructions for filling in the Declaration of Live Birth / Ministry of Health, Health Surveillance Secretariat, Department of Health Situation Analysis. - Brasília: Ministry of Health, 2011.

28-BRASIL. Secretariat of Health Surveillance. Department of Health Situation Analysis. Saúde Brasil 2010: an analysis of the health situation and selected evidence of the impact of health surveillance actions. Brasília, 2011.

29-Gravena AAF, Paula MGP, Marcon SS, CarvalhoMDB, PellososSM.Maternal age and factors associated with perinatal outcomes. Acta Paul Enferm. 2013; 26(2):130-5.

30-BRASIL. Secretariat of Health Care. Department of Primary Care. Low-risk prenatal care. Brasília: Ministry of Health, 2012a. (Primary Care Notebooks, n. 32).

31-Viellas EF etal.Prenatal care in Brazil. Cad. Saúde Pública, Rio de Janeiro, 30 Sup:S85-S100, 2014.

32-Viellas EF, Gama SGN, Theme Filha MM, Leal MC. Recurrent pregnancy in adolescence and negative outcomes in the newborn: a study in the municipality of Rio de Janeiro. RevBrasEpidemiol 2012; 15:443-54.

33-Leal MC, Gama SGN, Ratto KMN, Cunha CB. Use of the modified Kotelchuck index in the evaluation of prenatal care and its relationship with maternal characteristics and newborn weight in the municipality of Rio de Janeiro. Cad Saúde Pública 2004; 20 Suppl 1:S63-72. 28.

34-Domingues RMSM, Hartz ZMA, Dias MAB, Leal MC. Evaluation of the adequacy of prenatal care in the SUS network of the Municipality of Rio de Janeiro, Brazil. Cad Saúde Pública 2012; 28:425-37.

35-Coutinho T, Monteiro MFG, Sayd JD, Teixeira MTB, Coutinho CM, Coutinho LM. Monitoring the prenatal care process samongusers of the Unified Health Care System in a city of the Brazilian South east. RevBrasGinecolObstet 2010; 32:563-9. 6.

36-Ministry of Health.Consolidated Stork Network Ordinance. http://portal.saude.gov.br/portal/arquivos/pdf/portaria_consolidated_stork.pdf(accessed on 24/Sep/2016).

37-Santos MMAS, Baião MR, Barros DC, Pinto AA, Pedrosa PLM, Saunders C. Pre-gestational nutritional status, maternal weight gain, prenatal care conditions and adverse perinatal outcomes among adolescent puerperae. RevBras de Epidemiol, 2012;15(1):143-54.

38--Silva AAM etal.Neonatal near miss morbidity in the Nascer no Brasil survey.d. Saúde Pública, Rio de Janeiro, 30 Sup:S182-S191, 2014.

39-LEAL .M.C et al.Obstetric interventions during labour and delivery in Brazilian women at usual risk.Cad. Saúde Pública, Rio de Janeiro, 30 Sup:S17- S47, 2014.

40-Coimbra LC, Silva AAM, Mochel EG, Alves MTSSB, Ribeiro VS, Aragão VMF, et al. Factors associated with inadequate use of prenatal care. Rev Saúde Pública 2003; 37:456-62

41-Leal MC, Gama SGN, Campos MR, Cavalini LT, Garbayo LS, Brasil CLP, et al. Factors associated with perinatal morbidity and mortality in a sample of public and private maternity hospitals in the municipality of Rio de Janeiro, 1999-2001. Cad Saúde Pública 2004; 20 Supp 1:20-33.

42-Victora CG, Aquino EML, Leal MC, Monteiro CA, Barros FC, Szwarcwald CL. Maternal andchildhealth in Brazil: progressandchallenges. Lancet 2011; 377:1863-76.

43-Gama SGN etal.Factors associated with caesarean section among primiparous adolescents in Brazil, 2011-2012. Cad. Saúde Pública, Rio de Janeiro, 30 Sup:S117-S127, 2014.

44-D'Orsi E et al. Social inequalities and women's satisfaction with childbirth care in Brazil: a national hospital-based study. Cad. Saúde Pública, Rio de Janeiro, 30 Sup:S154-S168, 2014.

45-Barros AJD, Santos IS, Matijasevich A, Domingues MR, Silveira M, Barros FC, Victora CG. Patternsof deliveries in a Brazilianbirthcohort: almost universal cesareansections for thebetter-off. Rev Saúde Pública. 2011; 45 (4): 635-43.

46-Hansen AK, Wisborg K, Uldbjerg N, Henriksen TB. Risk of respiratory morbidity in term infants delivered by elective caesarean section: cohort study. BMJ 2008; 336:85-7.

47-CHAVES. R.L. Birth as a radical experience of change. Cad. Saúde Pública, Rio de Janeiro, 30 Sup:S14-S16, 2014.

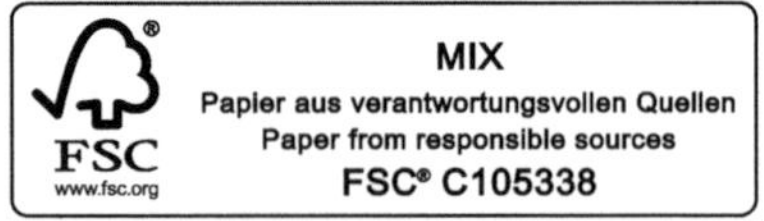

Printed by Books on Demand GmbH, Norderstedt / Germany